Yogini

Janice Gates

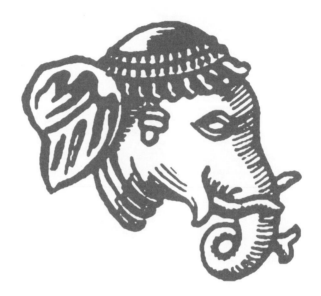

Yogini

The Power of Women in Yoga

Janice Gates

MANDALA
PUBLISHING

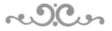

MANDALA
PUBLISHING

3160 Kerner Blvd. Unit 108
San Rafael, CA 94901
www.mandalapublishing.com
800.688.2218

Library of Congress Cataloging-in-
Publication Data available.

ISBN: 978-1932771-88-6

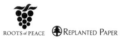

ROOTS of PEACE   REPLANTED PAPER

Roots of Peace is an internationally
renowned humanitarian organization
dedicated to eradicating landmines
worldwide and converting war-torn
lands into productive farms and wildlife
habitats. Together, we will plant 2 million
fruit and nut trees in Afghanistan and
provide farmers there with the skills and
support necessary for sustainable land use.

10 9 8 7 6 5 4 3 2

Cover image © 2004 Mahaveer Swami

Cover & Book Design: Michele Wetherbee
    & Iain Morris

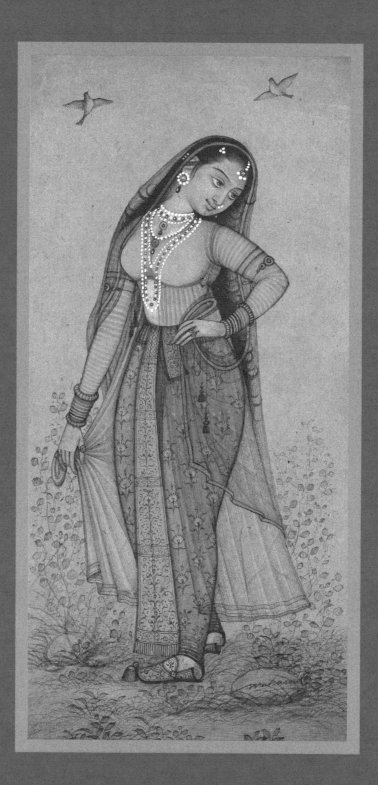

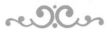

Table of Contents

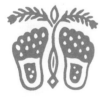

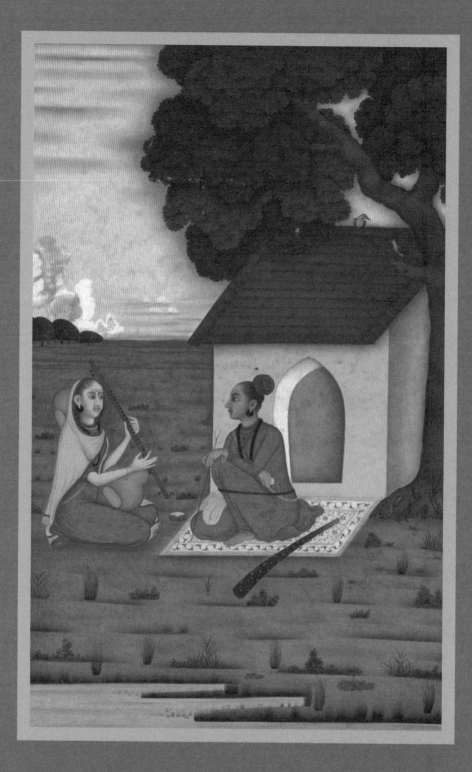

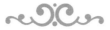

FOREWORD

by Linda Sparrowe

A few thousand years ago yoga, a mere whisper of a concept, began to emerge as a powerful vehicle for enlightenment. For men, that is. Sitting at the feet of their guru, these guys learned (and religiously practiced) what it took to prepare their bodies and minds for the rigors of meditation, which would ultimately liberate them from suffering.

Women on the other hand: not invited. And so it continued until 1937 when Indra Devi (fondly known as Mataji) convinced Krishnamacharya, one of the greatest yogis of modern times, to become her teacher. He, in turn, sent her out into the world to teach.

Despite Mataji's enormous popularity and her success bringing yoga to the masses, the masculine emphasis on physicality and rigorous discipline prevailed. We women flocked to male gurus and yoga teachers, unfolding our mats to learn the canon of asanas previously withheld. Before long we could execute difficult poses just as easily as a man could, and found a sense of power, equanimity, and discipline we had been searching for. But somewhere along the way, we lost the true spirit of yoga and a little of ourselves. Strengthening the body for sitting somehow became equated with

Opposite: Yogini with disciple, from West Bengal, India, 18th century.

learning harder and harder arm balances and inversions; discipline often took a nasty turn, as teachers controlled what students could and couldn't do in class and outside, too.

As more women began to teach, the face of yoga began to change, but that change didn't happen overnight. How could it have? Everything we had learned came from men; the advice we got from the scriptures was decidedly male-oriented—there's even a text that tells men what to do with their scrotums when practicing yoga but nothing that shows us what do to with our breasts! The language we used, the alignment cues we gave, the relationships we carved out with our students—that all came from our teachers. Every woman whose story Janice tells in this book owes a huge debt to at least one male teacher and freely honors his place in her life and in her teaching.

But luckily women have a way of bringing out the feminine aspects of anything we are passionate about, and yoga has proved to be no exception. At some point along her path, each of these women started to make the teachings her own. For some, the changes were subtle: softer language, different (gentler) metaphors, and new ways of explaining. It was the same practice, but with a different voice. For others, the need to break away proved irresistible, and they created their own unique brand of yoga.

No matter how these teachers redefined the path, today they appear united in their mission: to teach us what it means to be fully alive and truly at home with ourselves, and how to take the message of yoga out into the world. Yoga has always been about transformation and liberation.

Unfortunately, many women become fixated on the transforming part; that is, they think that by "transforming" their hips, thighs, breasts, or bellies, they'll find happiness. I like to think that the feminization of yoga starts with the premise that we are all perfect just the way we are. The transformation comes not in those hips and bellies, but in our attitudes about them as we learn to let go of (and thus become liberated from) society's dictates. We start on our yoga mats, but thanks to teachers like these, we take these concepts off the mat and into our everyday lives. We learn to see ourselves as we really are, without judgment, and embrace the power we have to enact change through kindness and compassion.

Yoga teaches us that out of small beginnings come great accomplishments, breath by breath, moment by moment. Think of a yoga class as a laboratory (or even a metaphor) for your life. It can teach you to recognize behaviors and patterns

in your life, encouraging you to let go of what doesn't work and embrace what does. Learning to stay in discomfort for ten breaths in a yoga pose may seem like a small beginning, but it can become a great accomplishment when you discover you can be in an uncomfortable situation in your life and not fall apart—for at least ten breaths. Indeed stepping onto your yoga mat is the first step in changing the world, because yoga has the power to change your relationship with yourself. It helps you to become friends with yourself, to make conscious and compassionate choices, and to pay attention to the outcome of those choices. This "small beginning" can indeed change the world, for if your yoga practice makes you a happier, calmer, and more present person, chances are the world you inhabit will be a happier, calmer place.

Over the years I've been blessed to call each of these women my teachers and many of them my friends. In their actions on and off the mat they have all reminded me of the true message of yoga written down in the Yoga Sutras centuries ago: act with discipline and compassion, reflect on those actions without judgment, and accept the outcome with loving curiosity. By thinking with my heart instead of my head, they say, I can bring the power of yoga to bear on the world's challenges, big and small. In fact, it is my duty as a woman and as a yogini to

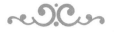

offer up the fruits of my yoga practice to benefit all living beings. I can start on my mat, paying attention to my own breath, carving out a loving relationship with my own body, but ultimately I can't be content just to practice yoga for myself; I must live it in everything I do. Yoga calls for a healthy dose of skillful action mixed with the right blend of open-mindedness, humor, and willingness. Put that all together and you have the means to discover the gifts you have to give. The next step is to move forward with clarity and compassion. Any of these women can help you do that. Read their stories. I guarantee they'll inspire you to take that next step.

LINDA SPARROWE has written numerous articles on women's health, herbs, and complementary medicine, as well as on yoga and Pilates. She is the former managing editor of *Yoga Journal* and is now a contributing editor. She is the author of several books, including *Yoga Journal*'s book, *Yoga*, featuring the beauty of yoga poses; and co-author, with Patricia Walden, of *The Woman's Book of Yoga and Health: A Lifelong Guide to Wellness*.

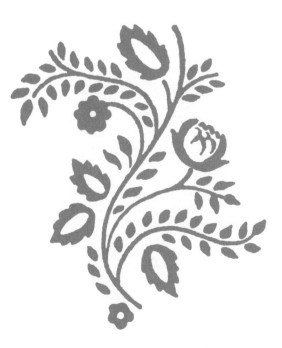

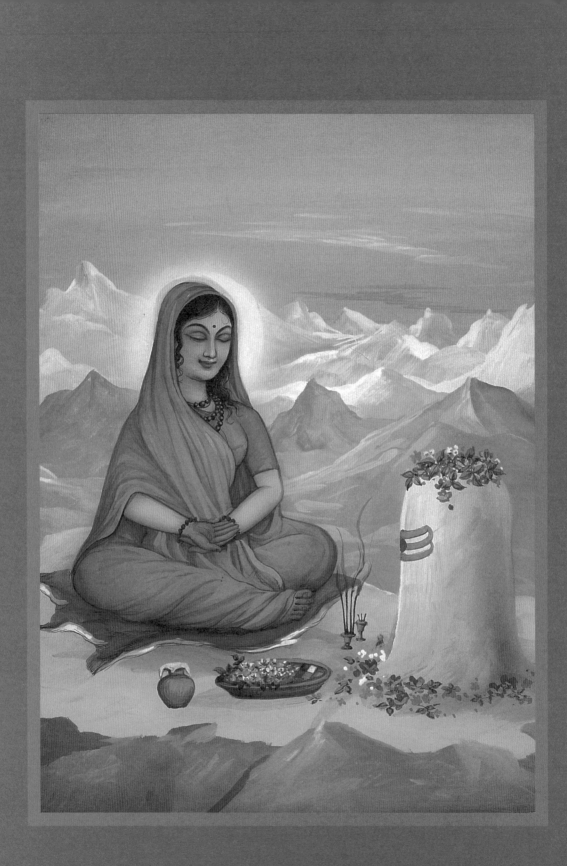

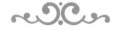

Introduction

For thousands of years, the deep river of women's wisdom has gone underground. It has been repressed, denied, and negated over centuries of patriarchy worldwide. In the United States today, the external chatter telling women how to look, what to buy, where to worship, what to do with our bodies is so loud that many of us no longer recognize who we truly are. Swept up in the current of a culture that values intellect over intuition, doing over being, repression over emotion, we lose contact with our own rhythms. We become too busy, we do too much. Losing this connection to our source, we dry up. How can we, as women, reconnect with our deep inner knowing? What is the path to revitalizing our spirit?

The teachings of yoga point the way home to reclaiming our female wisdom. Yoga is part of a spiritual practice which cultivates an awakening to our true Self. It is a vehicle for growth and development, whose ultimate goal is freedom from our limited perception of who we are and from the stories we allow to run and control our lives. The yoga postures we see today are

Opposite: The Hindu goddess and yogini Parvati is regarded as a representation of Shakti, the dynamic creative power inherent in reality.

only a small part of a vast tradition that includes overlapping—and sometimes conflicting—philosophies. But what they all have as their goal is *moksha*, liberation.

Yoga offers a path, a practice, and a way of life that honors the body, cultivates our vital life energy, and invites us to look closely at what binds us. The practice of yoga creates space for those outer voices to subside, so that we can tune in to what is true for us. Our lives don't suddenly become a seamless fairy tale where everything fits perfectly into place, but we learn to navigate our way with clear vision and deep inner knowing. We take time to turn our attention inward. We remember who we truly are, why we're here, and how to discover our personal path. As we slow down and return to our natural cycles, we can once again feel the rhythm of the universe and our place in it. That deep river comes back to life, winding, curving, ebbing and flowing, raging and subsiding.

The ancient spiritual traditions, including yoga, have come to us primarily through the words of men. Many women have been conditioned to accept this as the norm and perhaps unconsciously seek out masculine figures of authority or project our own inner knowing onto some outer image of the masculine Divine, God, or guru. Although the teachings themselves are universal and genderless, they have always been presented through a masculine filter. Most of the yoga texts were written, translated, and rewritten by men. As a result, the female perspective in yoga, as in most spiritual traditions, has been significantly underrepresented.

This book offers an opportunity to experience yoga through a new lens. You will get a glimpse of the original *yoginis* and luminaries who paved the way. And you'll meet inspiring women who are evolving the living practice of yoga to meet the needs of our culture and our time, like Rama Jyoti Vernon, whose global diplomacy offers a yogic model of how we can actualize our intentions in the outer world; Angela Farmer, who broke from tradition and form to develop her own unique approach to yoga; Nischala Devi, who spent eighteen years as a monk and pioneered programs integrating yoga with Western medicine; Sharon Gannon, whose in-your-face spirituality demands close examination of all our actions; Gurmukh Khalsa, who midwives women through their pregnancies with *kundalini* yoga; and Shiva Rea, a yogic river guide who reminds us, "Don't push the river, let it flow."

These *yoginis* have all come down from the mountain and integrated yoga into their daily lives. They are evolving the practice of yoga for women and men today and can serve as guides for our journey, encouraging us to look inside ourselves, to inquire within our own being, to find our own way. They are shaping and creating history in the spirit of the original yogis and yoginis. They balance their extensive study within the yoga tradition with their own experimentation. They stay close to their own hearts to find what is true for them. In the process, they empower other women to do the same and provide much-needed balance to the men who study and teach alongside them.

This book is the product of my own personal journey. My mother instilled feminist values in me: she made it clear that I could be anything and do anything, and that I didn't need a man to get there. I later discovered, however, that the internal barriers were set long ago, handed down over many generations and constantly reinforced in our modern culture. As I freely pursued my dreams as an adult— going to college, traveling, and studying— I continually sought external validation. I judged my body based on the idealized images in the media, and I doubted my decisions. In a world where practically every figure of authority was a man, I often looked to them for that validation, whether it was a teacher, father, or partner. Everywhere I turned, I found myself falling into the same old trap. So I kept moving.

At one point, I had read that meditation was the most direct path to peace and freedom. In search of these, I attended a ten-day silent meditation retreat in Thailand in 1989. By the third day, my entire body ached from sitting on the ground for hours at a time and I was exhausted from watching the endless stream of thoughts parading across the screen of my mind. I couldn't seem to find the "off" switch. That day, a woman offered a silent *hatha* yoga class, guiding us through gentle, flowing sun salutations. It was like a refreshing stream of cool water in the hot, dry environment of the monastery. Diving into my breath and my body, I began to feel my connection to the earth, the trees, and the sky. When I returned to sitting, rather than trying to control the movie in my mind, I felt myself opening to the vast space within and around me; I could no longer distinguish between what was me and what wasn't me. It felt like the entire universe was breathing through me, looking through my eyes. I was filled with an overwhelming sense of gratitude. As quickly as it came, this feeling left. I reverted right back to the feature film of my habitual thoughts. But I had a glimpse of what I had been seeking, and almost laughed out loud from the experience of how close it was. It became clear to me that the body was not something to be overcome or denied, but an integral part of remembering this wholeness.

Back home in the United States, I pursued my interest in yoga and meditation, and became a yoga teacher. But I found my old habits of trying to fit into an externally imposed ideal had hitched a ride. After striving to achieve a certain yoga pose, I ended up flat on my back with a low-back injury. There's nothing like an injury to give you that unexpected opportunity for reflection. Lying there, I began to question: Why practice yoga? Was I becoming more aware? Were my relationships more harmonious? Was I any closer to enlightenment? I realized that here I was, a Western woman in California, practicing a tradition that was originally taught to men by men through male lineages in India. Some very essential ingredient was missing in this union called yoga: the female experience. I wondered if I had to abandon my yoga practice or if there was another way.

Out of crises, solutions are born. In my case, this book was born. It began as a quest to uncover the history of women in yoga. But as I continued to practice and teach, I realized that the real story is about today's generation of women who have taken this male-dominated tradition and made it their own. While I researched women's historically limited participation in yoga and the oppressive social and cultural

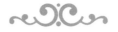

context out of which the yoga tradition arose, my classes and retreats continued to overflow with Western women.

Writing this book has given me immense insight into the oppressive history of women around the globe and the depth of the conditioning that is hardwired into our psyches. I discovered a new sense of urgency that is different from what motivated the feminist movement of the '60s—a revolution which made incredible and important progress for women. This book points to a new phase of the feminist revolution, an awakening from the conditioning that not only exploits and represses women, but also divides and separates women from men, and women from women. As yoga spreads in the West, it's easy to default to our deepest conditioning. Just a glance at the images of women in yoga magazines and advertisements tells volumes about the values that have been in place for so long. Is this the image of the enlightened feminine we want to model ourselves after? Coming back to the inspiring women in this book every day gives me immense hope that there is a better way.

The river of divine feminine wisdom has gone underground. I now realize that although hidden from view, it's not lost. It's my hope that in reading this book, you find inspiration and support to navigate

your way through the rapids, float for long stretches when there is no end in sight, read the current, and trust in that deeper pull to guide you.

May you feel this wonderful circle of women inviting you to come home to your true nature and remember who you are: powerful, peaceful, joyful, and free.

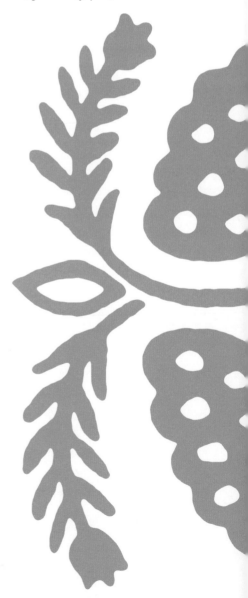

I went everywhere with longing
in my eyes, until here
in my own house

I felt truth
filling my sight.

–Lalla[1]

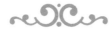

A History of Women in Yoga

YOGI OR YOGINI?
The oldest images resembling anything like the yoga we know today appear on soapstone seals found in the Indus Valley dating from around 3000 BCE. The figures on these seals, thought to be divinities in yogic postures, have stirred a spirited debate among scholars. Do they represent a female wearing multiple bracelets and a low slung belt, seated in Baddha Konasana? Or do they represent a male, seated on a throne, immersed in deep meditation?

Most scholars, being men, saw them as the latter. Others, primarily women, see them as the former. Interpretation is always limited by perception, as described by this graffiti, found on the wall below a mural of paintings of women in Sri Lanka (fourth century CE):

Don't we all see things our way?
For me, these women fly upward.
For you, they plunge from the sky.[2]

We may never know who this *yogini/yogi* was, or whether the figure was meditating, preparing for labor, or simply enjoying the beauty of nature. Considering the number of women practicing this posture in prenatal yoga classes today, however, it isn't difficult to imagine that some yoga postures were created by women, possibly in preparation for childbirth.

While images allude to one side of the story of women in yoga, the sacred texts of India reveal another: how the feminine was perceived in yoga philosophy. The inclusion of women in the study and teaching of yoga, and women's ability to chart their own spiritual destiny, changed over time. In early times, the sacred feminine was honored and earthly women revered, but for many centuries her divine image was overshadowed by male sky gods, and human women were devalued by elite priests and world-denying ascetics.

In much of the yoga tradition, which emphasized a philosophy of transcendence, the feminine principle was considered binding in her connection to nature and the material world. However, any energy that is relegated to the shadows for too long will eventually emerge to become illuminated and integrated, and the feminine principle in yoga is no exception. The feminine eventually returns in full force, opening new avenues for women in spiritual life, reminding us that "the immanent is pregnant with the transcen-

Opposite: A steatite seal of a divinity in a ritualized posture, from the Mohenjo-Daro region of ancient India, c. 1500 BCE.

dent,"[3] that it is right here, in the beauty and chaos of everyday life, that we can realize our true nature.

Although we don't know exactly when yoga first began, evidence of yogic practices and beliefs can be traced back to India's Indus Valley, where a highly developed civilization, revolving around the cites of Harappa and Mohenjo-Daro, thrived from around 2600 to 1900 BCE. Archeological remains found at excavation sites include large numbers of clay figurines of females, thought to be Mother Goddesses, wearing wide jeweled belts and multiple strands of necklaces. No weapons were unearthed. The picture that emerges from the ruins of this culture, a society called Harappan, is one of a relatively peaceful, female-oriented culture. It is here that we get our first glimpse of women in yoga.

It is believed that these early people practiced yoga in its widest sense, acknowledging the connection between the human and the divine realms through sacrificial rituals that may have centered on the fire ceremony. Women's inclusion in rituals was considered auspicious, even necessary, for the presence of the divine, and women were positively associated with fertility, growth, abundance, and prosperity. The spiritual guides of these ancient people were the *rishis*, or inspired "seers": men and women who, through meditative states, received visions and insights into the nature of reality, which they gave voice to in rhythmic poetry and symbolic language.

These hymnologic verses, known as the Rig Veda (knowledge of praise), served as a map to higher consciousness, and eventually became the first of four books that formed a vast collection of religious and philosophical incantations and instructions known as the Vedas (knowledge). More familiar yogic techniques, such as concentration, devotional invocation, recitation of hymns, breath control, and surrender of the ego (self-sacrifice) appear in the later Vedas: Sama Veda (knowledge of chant), Yajur Veda (knowledge of sacrifice), and Atharva Veda (knowledge of priests).

Some scholars believe that the oral tradition of the Vedas originated in the Indus Valley as far back as 5000 BCE. Others assert that this sacred literature arrived with Aryan tribes who migrated to the Indus Valley around 1500 BCE or earlier. Although we cannot be certain about the ultimate origins of the Vedas, we can confidently say that they show a continuity of symbolism and cultural motifs. Some of the female divinities of the indigenous culture influenced Vedic thought and were absorbed into the Vedic pantheon. The Rig Veda identifies Aditi, the goddess of creation, as the great womb into which the entire universe entered,

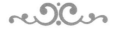

and states that all the male gods of the Vedas owe their birth to her. The goddess of the spoken word, Vac (speech), also appears. She represents divine intuitive knowledge and is considered the mother of the Vedas, sitting on the tongues of those chanting its sacred hymns. The seer Ambhrini (the one born of primeval ocean) is mystically identified with the goddess Vac, sometimes considered to be her mother. In realizing her own divine nature, Ambhrini sang ecstatically:

> *I am the sovereign queen . . .*
> *Creating all things, I blow forth like*
>   *the wind.*
> *Beyond heaven, beyond the earth am*
>   *I—so vast is my greatness.*[4]

The Vedas also contain the earliest written evidence of the position of women in religion. There are numerous references to female scholars, teachers, mystics, priestesses, and philosophers, and as many as twenty-seven female sages, including Lopamudra, a fully realized master whose husband was her disciple. Singing the hymns may have been the special expertise of women who were trained in music. In this tradition, a woman was free to study and become a *brahmacharini* (Vedic nun or ascetic) and the early forest universities were probably coeducational. Those women

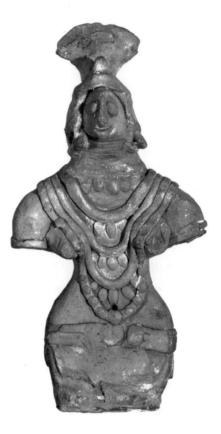

who did study were divided into two classes: *brahmavadinis*, lifelong students of philosophy and theology who pursued a solitary path, and *sadyodvahas*, women who studied and taught until they married. Teaching may actually have been a popular profession among women, who studied a wide range of subjects, including grammar, poetry, and literature as well as theology and philosophy.

Above: *Mother Goddess figurine, from Mohenjo-Daro c. 2600–1900 BCE.*

While the spiritual practice of the *rishis*, with its ritual and sacrifice, had a different flavor from the yoga we know today, it seems that these illumined sages, women among them, were already steeped in the spirit of yoga.

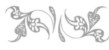

THE RISE OF THE BRAHMINS: THE FALL OF WOMEN

For reasons still debated among scholars, the status of women in religious life, and in society as a whole, diminished with the dramatic decline of the Indus civilization. This was a time of social and religious change that led to a gradual restructuring of society over many centuries. As the center of the culture moved east toward the fertile Gangetic Plains, a priestly class called the *brahmins* came into power and established a hierarchical religion called Brahmanism, which eventually became equated with Hinduism and led to a rigid caste system. The brahmins added their own commentaries on the Vedas, called the *Brahmanas* (c. 1000–800 BCE), which promoted a male-dominated worldview, particularly in the spiritual sphere. By the end of the Vedic period, this elite priesthood developed increasingly complex, exacting rituals and insular secret knowledge that was passed from father to son, ensuring patrilineal caste and patriarchal rule.

While the peasants in small villages continued to worship the goddess, Vedic society deemed earthly women impure. Aspects related to women's sexuality, such as menses, pregnancy, and birth—earlier associated positively with growth, abundance, and creation—became a phobic concern of the male priesthood. As the tension increased between a woman's inherent life-power, which infused the ritual with fertility, and her inherent impurity, which related to bleeding, her participation in ritual was increasingly limited.

Although yoga is not a religion, the history of women in yoga is inextricable from Hinduism and its influence on women's roles, particularly in relation to the social structure of the caste system with its four classes: the *brahmana* (priestly class) at the top, followed by *kshatriyas* (warriors), *vaishyas* (common people, such as merchants and artists), and finally, *shudras* (laborers). The top three classes were considered "twice born," as they enjoyed a physical birth followed by a ceremonial ritual birth: initiation into the Vedic tradition (*upanayana*), in which they received a sacred thread. Although originally both boys and girls participated in this ceremony, eventually females were no longer considered worthy of it.

In India, a land of esoteric teachings populated by yogis, mystics, wanderers, and poets, the nature of religion and philosophy was fluid and flexible with various traditions like Buddhism and Jainism integrating and overlapping—even those with conflicting views. While many of these religions revered the feminine in her celestial form and honored the feminine qualities related to motherhood, such as selflessness and servitude, male gods reigned, and embodied women were viewed negatively, particularly in relation to their biology.

It is interesting to note that as women were subjugated worldwide in patriarchal cultures, they had less authority in religion than in any other sphere. The once vital feminine principle seemed to be sinking into the shadowy recesses of the collective psyche.

PRECLASSICAL YOGA: WHERE ARE THE WOMEN?

As the Brahmanic faith became excessively ritualistic and exclusive, around the sixth century BCE, a new set of spiritual practices arose based on texts called the Upanishads (meaning "to sit near," as with a teacher). We get a last glimpse of the public participation of women in religion in the early Upanishads with the female philosopher Gargi, who boldly challenged the sage Yajnavalkya in a pivotal debate at the court of King Janaka on the nature of the true self. After that, mention of women in the spiritual texts continues to wane.

What many consider to be the seeds of yoga became a full-fledged spiritual tradition in the divinely inspired texts of the Upanishads. In the Upanishads, the focus shifted from the external ritual of the Vedas to internal spiritual practices, whose aim was to realize that our innermost essence, *Brahman* (the self), is the same as the essence of the universe, *atman* (or soul, also called *purusha*). According to Vedanta, the philosophical system based on the teachings of the Upanishads, there exists only one principle: Brahman. Everything else, including what we perceive as the material world, is brought about by *maya*, the illusory feminine force which veils the true knowledge of the underlying unity of reality. As *maya*, the feminine principle is a creative power of differentiation, but in Vedanta she is also equated with ignorance and delusion, which must be overcome to attain liberation.

The concept of *karma* (action) also arose in these texts, with the sense that actions in this lifetime determine the nature of rebirth. This was further developed into the belief that through intense meditation and renunciation, *karma* could be transcended, thus ending the cycle of reincarnation. For many, this implied transcending the human condition, rather than being entangled in its illusory dream. Transcendence could be taken literally, meaning to leave everyday life for a solitary existence, or symbolically, meaning to let go of all attachments, including the ego. Most men on the spiritual path headed for the caves and forests for a life of renunciation, while most women stayed home and tended the fire.

The life of an ascetic involved wandering alone and was not considered practical or safe for a woman, who would be unprotected, vulnerable, and considered unchaste. The Upanishads stressed *jnana* yoga (the path of knowledge), which further limited women, who had become associated with ignorance in the Brahmanas. In addition, a woman's connection to the physical body, with its monthly bleeding and birth-related fluids, connected her to impurity. In many cases, she was viewed as an evil seductress who could or might lure a man away from his highest calling.

By this time, women were being married off at the prepubescent age of ten to ensure their purity. Where previously sons and daughters were equally welcomed, females became a liability to the family due to the dowry system, which calls for the bride to be accompanied by a financial gift to the husband's family. Women were

valued for their chastity and purity, rather than their education or intelligence, and yet their lack of education led to the view that they were ignorant and incapable in the religious sphere outside of the home. The possibilities for women narrowed until their restricted roles as dutiful wife and mother solidified.

As the priestly class that dominated Vedic culture and religion subjugated women in the last centuries of the pre-Christian era, the *Manava Dharma Shastra* (*Laws of Manu*) carried this process even further. Compiled around 200 BCE, the 2,685 verses of the *Laws of Manu* spelled out the *dharma* (doctrine), or social obligations and duties of the various castes and individuals—primarily addressing "twice born" men during the four stages of life: student, householder, forest-dweller, and ascetic. Women were ascribed one phase, the *stridharma*, or householder phase. After a man had completed the householder phase of his life, he was to head off to a forest hermitage and could either leave his wife under the protection of their sons or take her with him. For the final phase of life, he was to "abandon this foul-smelling, tormented, impermanent dwelling place of living beings, filled with urine and excrement"[5] and wander as an

_____

Opposite: *An ascetic hanging over a fire.*

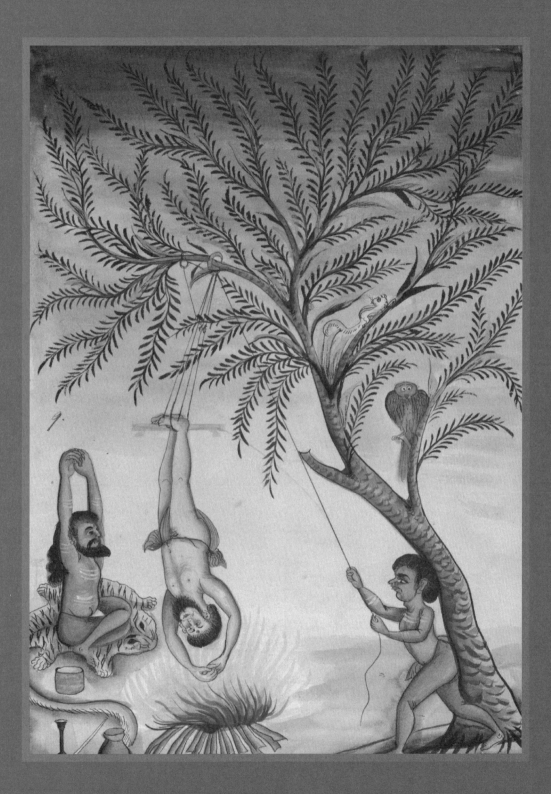

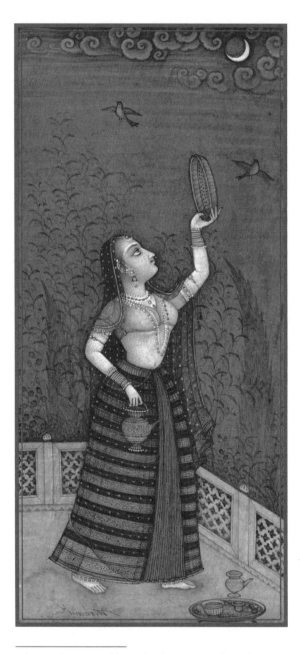

Above: The river goddesses (Such as Ganga, shown here) represent the free-flowing movements of consciousness and its creative energy—uninhibited, purifying, and clarifying.

ascetic—alone. A combination of legal injunctions and moral prescriptions, the text speaks for itself:

> A virtuous wife should constantly serve her husband like a god, even if he behaves badly, freely indulges his lust, and is devoid of any good qualities.[6]

> The bed arid, the seat, jewelry, lust, anger, crookedness, a malicious nature, and bad conduct are what Manu assigns to women.[7]

While the essence of the Upanishadic teachings spoke to the possibility for *moksha*, or liberation in the here and now, what was the most women could hope for? To be reborn as a man.

During this time, outside of and parallel to the Vedic religion, other tribal religions with their own spiritual practices, gods, and goddesses, continued to thrive. While male deities dominated the Vedic pantheon as a reflection of their patriarchal culture, at all other levels of society, the chosen deity was the *grama devata*, the local village goddess who presided over the welfare of the village, echoing back to the time of the *rishis* in the Indus Valley. As Brahmanism began its steady decline, in part due to the rise of Buddhism and Jainism, these popular religions began to assert themselves.

The Gita's Yoga

The Bhagavad Gita (Lord's Song), which appeared in the middle of the first millennium BCE, introduced the idea that everyone—including women—could participate in spiritual life. This text arose from Vaishnavism, a religion centered on worshipping the divine in the form of Vishnu, specifically in his incarnation as Krishna. Part of a larger epic (the Mahabharata), the Bhagavad Gita takes place on a battlefield as a dialogue between the warrior Prince Arjuna and Lord Krishna. The yoga of the Gita still promoted *jnana* yoga, but began to reconnect spiritual practice with daily life through *karma* yoga and *bhakti* yoga (devotional yoga). Unlike the Upanishadic view, the Gita emphasized freedom in action, that to reach enlightenment, it's not our actions that we must renounce (in fact, those are important as part of our social obligations), but it is the fruit of those actions we must surrender.

The integral yoga of the Gita built a bridge between the previously exclusive Vedic teachings and the wider culture, through *bhakti* yoga, which brought the teachings out of the dry, impersonal, abstract realm into the lived experience of the people; from the head to the heart.

This was the beginning of a larger *bhakti* yoga movement, which would later become one of the most popular spiritual practices available to women. However, before *bhakti* yoga fully flowered, yoga was systematized in Patanjali's Yoga Sutras.

Classical Yoga: Patanjali's Yoga Sutras

Possibly the most familiar text on yoga today, the Yoga Sutras are a collection of 196 aphorisms codified by the sage Patanjali around 200 CE that form an outline or systematic guide to the practice of yoga. Patanjali promoted the eight-limbed path known as *raja* yoga (royal yoga), which includes the moral and ethical principles foundational to spiritual practice, instructions on meditation, and teachings on liberation. This path also promotes a view of existence that is a radical departure from the nondual philosophy of the Upanishads.

Patanjali is aligned with the ideal of Classical Sankhya, a school of thought which promulgates existence as two primordial, interdependent principles: *purusha*, pure consciousness, which is male, and *prakriti*, nature incarnate, which is female. Spirit and matter, joined as one in the Upanishads, are separated here. This yoga, often referred to as Classical Yoga, acknowledges the dynamic role of the feminine principle, *prakriti*, literally defined as "she who brings forth," in her ever-changing appearance as everything manifest. *Purusha* is the seer; *prakriti*, the seen. The purpose of yoga is to move from identification with the seen back into the pure consciousness of the seer—experienced as the continuous enjoyment of infinite bliss. *Prakriti* is composed of three basic *gunas* (qualities)—*sattva* (purity/joy), *rajas* (activity/passion), and *tamas* (lethargy/dullness), which are considered the three components of materiality that bind us to the sensual world (*guna* literally means "rope"). For the transcendent quality of *purusha* to shine through, a seeker must withdraw their attachment to these qualities inherent in nature.

Thus, the feminine principle of *prakriti* is both liberating and binding. She is endlessly creative, but ties one to the material world through the *gunas*. While the teachings of Classical Yoga themselves aren't gender-specific, their interpretation and application reflected the social values of the time. The bias towards the *sattvic* state, which was equated with the natural state of the mind and its ability to reflect pure consciousness, was not favorable to women, who were associated with the characteristics of *tamas* and *rajas*.

Although not a path of complete renunciation (the Yoga Sutras included elements of devotion and *karma* yoga), in keeping with the spirit of the times, Patanjali's emphasis was on transcending the human condition, and conditioning through concentration, meditation, and *tapas*, austerities that create an "inner heat" that creates the desired transformation of consciousness.

Where were women now? The status of women during this time reflected their position in a male-dominated culture, particularly with the Laws of Manu defining women's position solely in relation to men—first her father, then her husband, and finally her sons. A woman's worth was still connected to her loyalty, chastity, docility, and strength, which arose out of *tapas*. Feminine self-sacrifice is a common model of women's religiosity in most patriarchal religions and is taken to the extreme in the case of Hindu women. For example, if a Hindu woman's husband died first, she was encouraged to perform *sati*, immolating herself on his funeral pyre.

While many Hindu women may have had their spiritual yearnings satisfied by incorporating male religion into their domestic world, many clearly did not. Evidence exists that not everyone followed

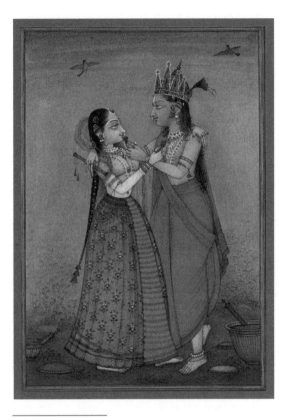

the *Laws of Manu*. Inscriptions by women dating to the first and second centuries BCE have been found on monuments, indicating that women held property and were free to spend their wealth as they wished. There is also some contradiction within the various texts. While Manu denied women education, the *Amarakosa*, a text dating from the fourth century, lists *acharyas* and *upadhyayis*, female religious instructors and teachers, indicating that some women were educated. Finally, while most of the spiritual texts and teachings give only the worldview of the elite, educated males of the culture, the images of Tantra allude to another side of the story.

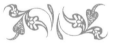

Above: *Radha and Krishna, two lovers personifying the dual forces Nature (prakriti) and Pure Consciousness (purusha), who sustain the universe.*

TANTRA: REEMERGENCE OF THE FEMININE

Side by side with these ascetic traditions, Tantra flourished underground. In complete opposition to Brahmanism, Tantra was a reversal of the ascetic view: all that was mysterious, feared, and controlled by the Brahmins became sacred in Tantra. Rather than seeing bodily existence as an illusory obstacle to overcome on the path to enlightenment, Tantra viewed it as a delightful manifestation of *Shakti*, the divine feminine power in her multitude of forms, that offered a vehicle for enlightenment. In the Tantric texts, women are revered as representations of *Shakti* and accepted not only as practitioners, but as teachers.

Spreading in small rural communities, Tantra is said to have come forward in the middle of the first millennium CE to serve the needs of those living in the *kali yuga*, the dark age filled with greed, ignorance, and delusion. The body, in other traditions considered "a putrid heap of flesh and bones," became a temple of the Divine: celebrated, honored, even enjoyed! A religion of the masses, Tantra tore down class and gender barriers in the spiritual arena, making enlightenment an option for all who were willing and able. This revolutionary spirituality taught that enlightenment was not to be found anywhere other than here and now in this life—exactly as it is.

A precursor of hatha yoga (described below), Tantra viewed the body as a microcosm of the entire universe; within each person the universal energy, *shakti*, sleeps coiled at the base of the spine in the form of *kundalini*, the serpent energy. The practices of *asana, pranayama, mudra,* and *bandha* were designed to awaken and direct this energy through the *chakras*, psychospiritual centers, uniting *shakti* with *shiva* at the crown of the head. Under the guidance of a guru, the adept learned the use of *mantras* (sacred sounds), *yantras* (geometric diagrams), rituals, visualizations, and meditation to realize the unity of the inner self and the outer universe.

Central to the Tantric practices is the invocation of the feminine principle, and in this way Tantra is closely related to Shaktism, the Hindu goddess tradition that originates with the goddess-worshipping culture of the Indus Valley. In the Shakta tradition, the mother of the universe, Devi (meaning "shining one"), is said to have come to shine her light on the ignorance and delusion that has plagued our world. In the Shakta text, as the Devi-Mahatmya (glorification of the goddess), she is worshipped as the feminine in all her forms: gentle and loving, but also fierce, powerful, and terrifying. Various concepts of the feminine principle (*prakriti, maya, shakti*) come together in the Devi Mahatmya to create a Great Goddess who is the power inherent in creation and dissolution; formless yet the matrix of all forms; immanent and transcendent.

Shaktism is not exclusive to women; some of the most revered saints of modern times were shaktas, including Ramakrishna, Swami Vivekananda, Paramahansa Yogananda, and Sri Aurobindo.

> In Shaktism God (Shiva) is the silent unmoving one over whose prostrate body the Goddess rampages; she (Shakti) is dynamic, self-willed

---

Opposite: Sodashi is one of the Mahavidyas (wisdom goddesses) representing the independent, powerful, and fearsome aspects of the divine feminine.

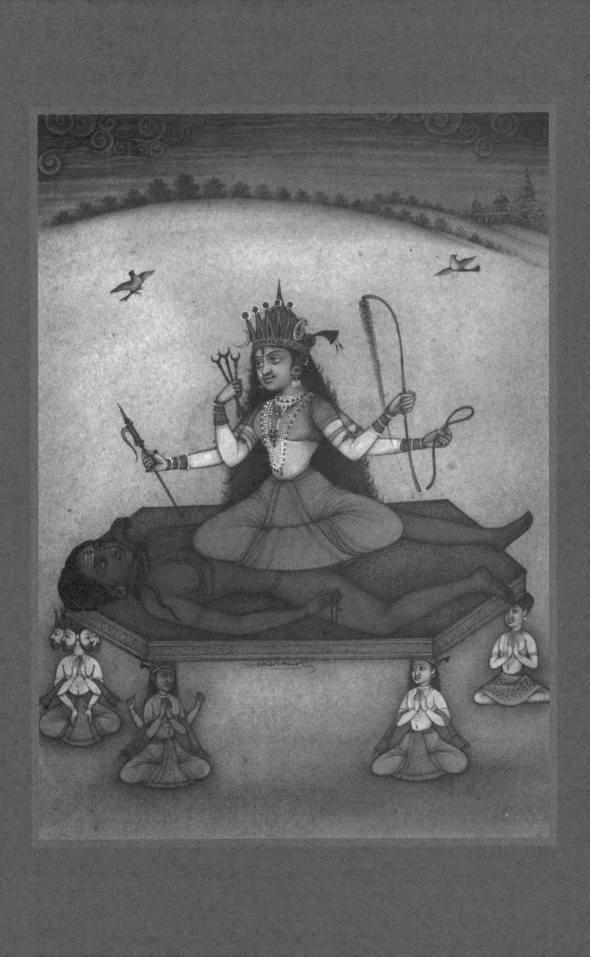

energy. And then again, the Goddess is the primordial unchanging universal awareness which enjoys the swirling movements of her beloved, Shiva Nataraja, whose dance of creation and destruction begins and ends world systems. God and Goddess interchange active and passive roles like lovers, unrestricted by human definitions.[8]

Female adepts of yoga and practitioners of Tantric lore were called *yoginis*: women who renounced societal norms in search of spiritual knowledge through the practice of yoga. Legends and tales about yoginis tell of their *siddhis*, or supernatural powers, acquired through long years of practice, ranging from extraordinary wisdom to being able to fly through the air or transform people into animals or birds. In Mughul and Rajput paintings from the eighteenth century, these yoginis are portrayed as ascetics with disciples. They are also portrayed as having powers over animals.

The ancient yogini has many faces in Indic culture: she is portrayed as a female ascetic, a sorceress, a witch, or an attendant to the goddess. Devi herself is sometimes referred to as *Mahayogini*, the Great Yogini, a form of the supreme goddess of the shaktas.

Texts that refer to the more esoteric cults of yoginis reveal little, emphasizing the highly secretive nature of the teachings, which were only divulged to initiates. However, images of yoginis carved into temples have inspired research into their ritual practices.

Yoginis were associated with the Kaula sect of Tantra which subscribes to non-Brahmanic practices known as the five Ms: *mamsa* (meat), *matsya* (fish), *mudra* (parched grain), *madya* (wine), and *maithuna* (sexual intercourse). The Kaula rituals took place in the elaborate circular yogini temples and ranged from sacrificing animals to worshipping goddesses in symbolic form as *chakras* on cloth. In the *maithuna* (sexual) ritual, the yogini, as the earthly representation of Shakti, received the male as the earthly equivalent of Shiva.

While some people confuse Tantra with an "anything goes" philosophy and wild sex, even the practices of the most esoteric sects had symbolic significance. In the Tantric cosmology, *viparita-rati* (sexual union with the female partner in the superior position) is symbolic of the feminine principle constantly aspiring to create unity from duality.

Shakti (the creative dynamic principle) and Shiva (the male principle of pure consciousness) are often shown embracing or dancing together. Theirs is the dance between freedom and limitation, spirit and matter, body and mind. It is this interplay of the archetypal male and female principles that gives rise to the entire cosmos. It is because of the interplay of life and matter that nature is able to reveal itself in all its glory.

In Shaktism women and men are not at war, but through their collective uniqueness realize the feminine fullness of the universe. They are the images on earth of the unitary cosmic principle, and in imbalance, they disturb the macrocosmic equilibrium. The two must be in one male-female relationship in order, as Vivekananda put it, to 'restore the essential balance in the world between the masculine and feminine energies and qualities. The bird of the spirit of humanity cannot fly with one wing.'[9]

Tantra revived the prepatriarchal values of nature, creation, sexuality, and the feminine, which had been surviving on the fringes of Brahmanic culture.

During this revolutionary period when new doors to spiritual life were opening for women, some continued to thrive in the home, while others left. One such woman, the Kashmiri yogini and poet Lalleshvari, known as Lalla, left an unhappy marriage

and is known for wandering and dancing naked as she sang her songs—reminiscent of the ancient *rishis*:

You are the sky and the ground.
You alone the day, the night air.
You are all things born into being.[10]

Lalla's poetry reveals her Tantric leanings as well as her knowledge of the technology of yoga:

Some people abandon their homes.
Others abandon hermitages.
All this renunciation does nothing,
     if you're not deeply conscious.
Day and night, be aware
     with each breath,
     and live there.
My teacher, you are God to me!
Tell me the inner meaning
     of my two breathings,
     the one warm, the other cool.
In your pelvis near the navel is the source
     of many motions called the sun,
     the city of the bulb.
As your vitality rises from that sun, it
     warms and in your mouth it meets
     the downward flow through the
     fontanelle of your higher self, which
     is cool and called the moon, Shiva.
This rivering mixture feels,
     by turns, warm and cool.[11]

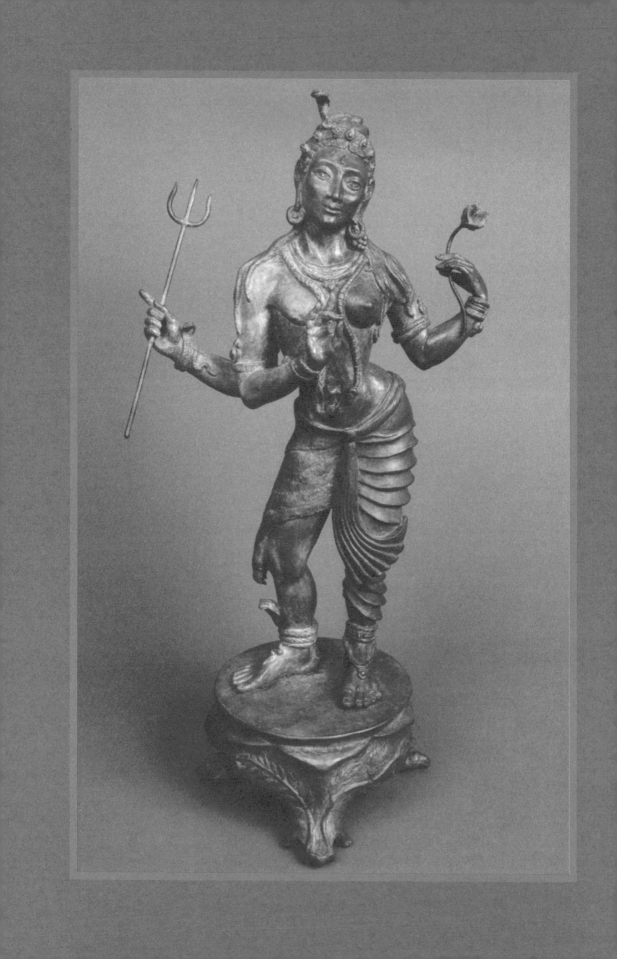

Although few today practice Tantra the way it was originally practiced, we can see its influence in *hatha* yoga, and there has been a contemporary revival of a certain type of Tantra called Kashmir Shaivism whose main principles have been spread in the West by people like Gurumayi Chidvilasananda.

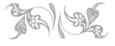

Bhakti Yoga: Yoga of the Heart

With the return of the feminine principle in yoga philosophy and practices, Tantra created fertile soil for *bhakti* yoga (the yoga of devotion), which first sprouted in the yoga of the Bhagavad Gita, and fully blossomed around 900 CE. *Bhaktas* (devotees) on the path of *bhakti* yoga seek to dissolve the ego into the divine, focusing and directing their emotional energy towards a god or goddess until mystical union is achieved. For many, worshipping the divine through singing, dancing, and meditation offered a middle path between extreme asceticism and the radical practices of Tantra. Rather than negating or attempting to transcend human feelings and emotions, *bhakti* yoga validates and engages them as powerful tools for achieving enlightenment. For women, *bhakti* yoga was especially attractive because suddenly they could give voice to their spiritual experience outside of the home through singing and love-intoxicated chanting. Since the ideal type of devotion in this system was not to the husband as her lord, but exclusively to god, some women, in radical defiance of societal norms, refused to marry or left their husbands altogether. The ecstatic, devotional spirit of *bhakti* yoga echoes back to the early *rishis*.

There were numerous female *bhakti* saints who were mystical poets who praised the divine, including Mirabai, an educated woman who left her prince-husband to wander in passionate dedication to her Lord Giridhara.

> *O friend, understand: the body*
> *is like the ocean,*
> *rich with hidden treasures.*
> *Open your innermost chamber and*
> *light its lamp.*
> *Within the body are gardens,*
> *rare flowers, peacocks, the inner*
> *Music; on it the white soul swans*
> *take their joy.*

Opposite: Shiva/Shakti, also known as Ardhanarishwara. The half-male, half-female deity symbolizes the integrated unity of opposites. (Sculpture by Patricia Sullivan.)

And in the body, a vast market—
    go there, trade, sell yourself for a
    profit you can't spend.
Mira says, her Lord is beyond praising.
Allow her to dwell near Your feet.[12]

Probably the best known female saint today is Amritanandamayi Ma, known as Ammachi, who since childhood has been absorbed in devotion. She is considered the embodiment of unconditional love. With no formal training or guru, she travels the world teaching love by being love. Known as the "hugging guru" she embraces the masses with open arms, attracting thousands.

Today, American musicians Deva Premal, Jai Uttal, and Krishna Das continue the devotional tradition of *kirtan* (chanting), another form of *bhakti* yoga. Through call-and-response group chanting, these artists draw crowds of blissed-out Western yogis and yoginis seeking a way to link with the divine.

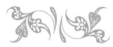

HATHA YOGA: EMBODIED BEINGS

How do all of these ancient texts and esoteric practices relate to the yoga we see today—the pretzel-like postures being taught in gyms, recreation centers, and yoga studios around the world? The yoga postures and breathing practices most familiar to us have their roots in the psychospiritual technology of Tantra. However, like much of yoga, the beginnings of hatha yoga are shrouded in mystery, as the tradition was originally passed down orally. The Hindu tradition associates the creation of hatha yoga with Gorakshanath, an eleventh-century realized adept who is said to have founded *kanphata*, hermits and monastic groups consisting of people from the lower classes, many of whom were women. Gorakshanath's teacher, Matsyendranath, is said to have founded the Yogini Kaula school, out of which the Yogini cult (described earlier) is thought to have emerged.

With this background, it's no surprise that hatha yoga expresses Tantric ideals, which recognize that the ecstatic experience of enlightenment is a full-body event. The physical practices of hatha yoga were designed to prepare the body for this powerful experience, which can have profound effects on the body and the nervous system. The cleansing techniques, yoga postures, breathing practices, seals, and locks help balance and mobilize the life force sleeping at the base of the spine (*kundalini shakti*), which can then ascend to the crown for the microcosmic marriage of *shiva* and *shakti*. The term *hatha* itself is esoterically explained as the union between *ha*, the solar force, and *tha*, the lunar force. To balance and unite these opposing forces takes substantial effort, which explains why hatha yoga was originally called the "yoga of force."

While many hatha yoga texts exaggerate the benefits of practice—claiming you will live forever if you do this and die if you do that—they point to the underlying truth that the physical body eventually disintegrates. What remains cannot die. The exaggerated claims also act as warnings to practice under an experienced teacher. Although written by men for men, the *Hatha Yoga Pradapika*, the *Gheranda-Samhita*, and the *Shiva-Samhita*, composed somewhere between the late thirteenth and early eighteenth centuries, do include references to female energy. Early texts refer to the symbolic intermingling of male and female semen as the realization that all that appears separate is actually united. The references to the *yoni* (vagina) and *lingam* (phallus) in the *Hatha* yoga texts point to the eternal play between the feminine power and masculine consciousness, which are experienced as separate on the relative level but are always united in the absolute.

Some texts do mention women, like the *Yoga Yajnavalkya* (c. 1200 CE), which is written as a dialogue between Yajnavalkya and his wife Gargi. This text implies that

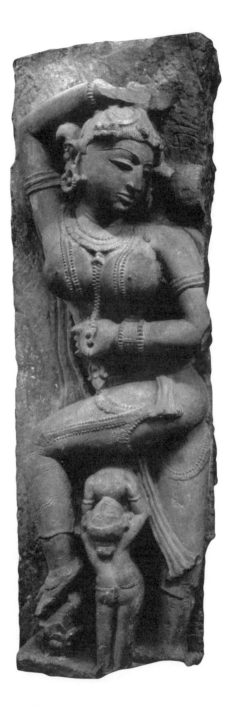

Above: *Female displaying yogic twist, from Kajuharo Museum.*

yoga is open to both men and women, but simultaneously prohibits women from certain practices, like using the mantra "om." The *Yoga Rahasya*, attributed to Sri Nathamuni (c. 850 CE), also has practices for women, particularly for pregnancy.

Although the yoga postures were originally thought to have been practiced only by men, common images in post-eighth-century art suggest otherwise, as images of female bodies in yogic-like twists abound in north Indian sculpture. The *devadasis*, early Indian temple dancers whose playful images adorn temples, also hint at the practice of yoga as part of their dance. One yogini-scholar, Roxanne Kamayani Gupta, suggests that as the wild, ecstatic forms of Tantra went underground, the more acceptable figure of the yogini as the living goddess, or Mother, known as Amma or Mataji, became popular. In the same way, *devadasis* may have replaced the early yoginis as ritual specialists and symbols of feminine power. Even today, *asanas* are considered foundational to classical Indian dance, which is practiced by women and men alike.

While many of the practices in the early texts may seem esoteric to the modern reader, they all have at their root the same goal: a return to the source of consciousness, which ultimately resides in the heart. And it is this that attracts people to yoga today.

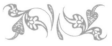

YOGA COMES WEST

One of the earliest women to bring the teachings of yoga to the West was a cigar-smoking occultist, the Russian immigrant Madame Blavatsky. In 1875, along with Colonel Henry Steel Olcott, a prominent New York lawyer, she founded the Theosophical Society to promote Eastern esotericism in the West. *Isis Unveiled* (1877) and *The Secret Doctrine* (1888), her books on the secret teachings of the Vedas and Upanishads, captivated American readers. A steady stream of Indian swamis followed, beginning with Swami Vivekananda, who introduced thousands of people to *Raja* yoga at the Parliament of World Religions in Chicago in 1893.

The current manifestation of yoga, with its focus on postures and breathing practices, can be traced back to a few teachers in India. The ones who have most notably influenced women are Swami Sivananda Saraswati and T. Krishnamacharya. Swami Sivananda was one of the first to initiate women into *sanyas* (monas-

Opposite: Yogini Sharon Gannon, whose story begins on page 67.

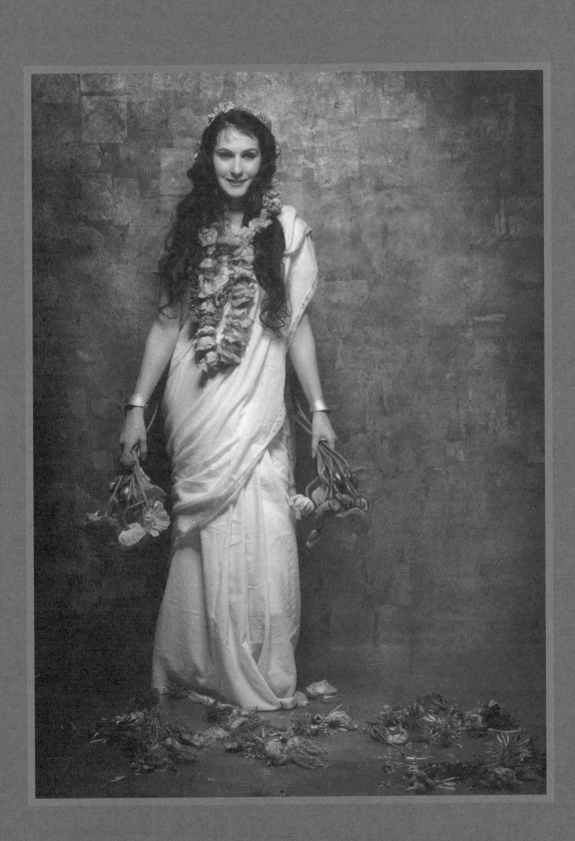

tic life) and through his lineage women like Lilias Folan, Nischala Devi, and Swami Radha (all profiled in this book) spread yoga in the West. He offered a gentle hatha yoga practice as a complement to his Integral Yoga approach that synthesized *karma, jnana,* and *bhakti* yogas.

If you walk into a yoga class today, what you see most often has some connection to the yogi-scholar T. Krishnamacharya and his students. In an attempt to revive yoga from its decline in the beginning of the twentieth century, Krishnamacharya toured all over India, giving lectures and demonstrations, not realizing that his teachings would spread throughout the world without him ever leaving his native land. It was through his students—most notably a Western woman, Indra Devi—that his yoga became known outside his home country. He also taught Mary Louise Skelton, who brought his teachings to Colgate University in central New York state. Krishnamacharya's teaching of women may have been influenced by his own teacher of more than seven years, Rama Mohana Brahmachari, who lived in a remote cave in Tibet with his wife and three children. In return for teaching, Brahmachari asked Krishnamacharya to pass on the teachings of yoga, not as a renunciate in a cave, but in a way that could benefit modern householders.

Although it wasn't considered appropriate at the time, it appears that Brahmachari himself taught yoga to women. There is a small book of illustrations Krishnamacharya passed on to his son, TKV Desikachar, showing yoga postures drawn by Brahmachari's daughter. Half of these illustrations are of men and half of women. Krishnamacharya also taught his wife Namagiriamma and his sister-in-law Jayammal. Later in life, Krishnamacharya regarded women as superior to men in terms of yoga and felt they were going to preserve the tradition.

Other students of Krishnamacharya's have been influential in spreading hatha yoga to the West and to women. BKS Iyengar, Krishnamacharya's brother-in-law, known for his precise alignment and use of props, taught many women, including his daughter, Geeta Iyengar, who focused on yoga for women and wrote *Yoga: A Gem for Women* in 1990. Other notable students of BKS Iyengar include Patricia Walden, whose image is one of the most recognizable in the yoga world today because of her yoga videos, and Vanda Scaravelli, who met Iyengar at her summer villa in Switzerland at the age of forty-five and started daily yoga lessons with him. Scaravelli also later studied with Desikachar and went on to become one of the most inspiring teachers in the West.

The popular power and *vinyasa* yoga classes that fill yoga centers and gyms alike is linked to Sri K. Pattabhi Jois, who further developed the ashtanga vinyasa yoga that he learned from Krishnamacharya. Krishnamacharya's son, Desikachar, had a wide view of his father's teaching, particularly its emphasis on yoga for healing. Desikachar has taught many Western women, including Sonia Nelson, profiled in this book.

Yoga has indeed come full circle. This ancient tradition, which emerged from a goddess-worshipping culture and was subsequently hidden from women, is now experiencing a major resurgence in India, primarily due to the popularity of hatha yoga in the West. Today, yoga is being revitalized all across Asia, in many cases by women.

There are currently over sixteen million people practicing yoga in the United States, almost eighty percent of whom are women. Many of these contemporary yoginis around the globe are making a truly valuable contribution to this evolving tradition, as they have become less focused on form and structure and are now balancing their yoga with an intuitive, inner-guided practice, rather than one that meets outer ideals. They are emphasizing the importance of integrating spiritual practice into our day-to-day activities and interactions.

Yoga is a living and evolving tradition, which, as with most spiritual wisdom traditions, must be tested in the laboratory of one's own body, mind, and heart—just as millions of modern women are doing today. The women profiled in this book speak to the many challenges, insights, and epiphanies we may encounter along the way.

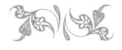

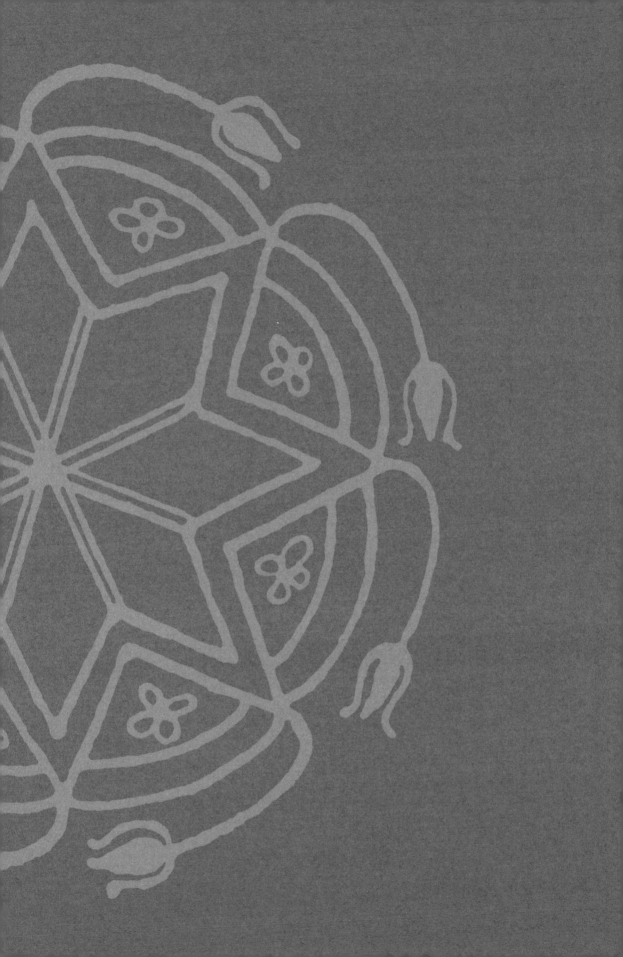

Yoginis

ONE OCEAN, MANY RIVERS

When sleeping women wake,
mountains move.

–Chinese proverb

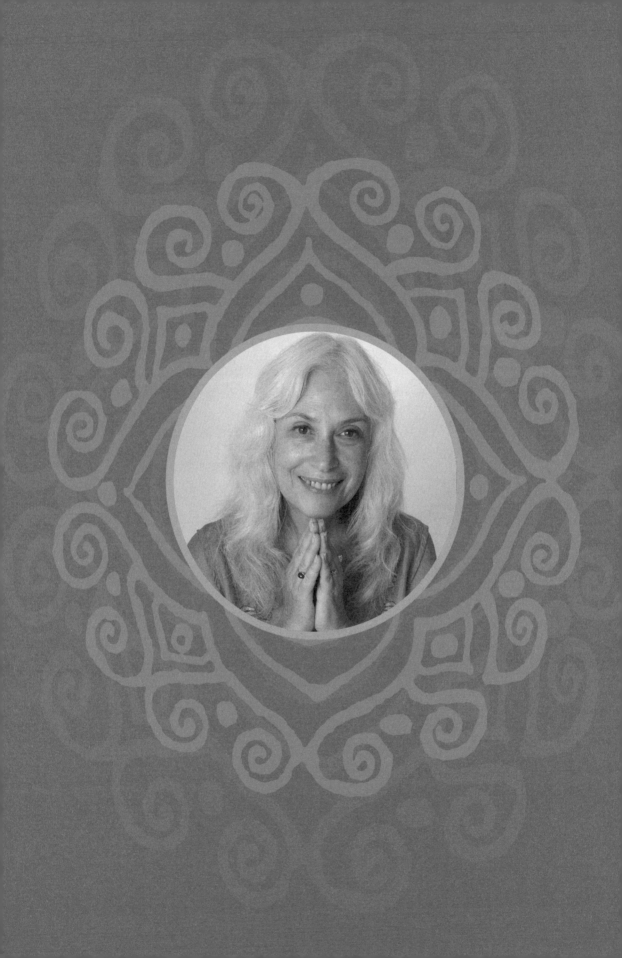

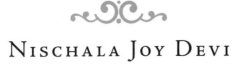

Nischala Joy Devi

No matter what you do, you see your body
change. No matter what you do, no matter how
conscious you are, the body gets older.
You can't stop it. If all yoga practice is focused
on the body, and it is not able to effect the
changes, you might become frustrated and sad.
Instead, if you know that you are the
Divine being living within the body, then no
matter how the body looks or feels,
you know that you are the ever-present
unchanging Divine.

High up in the hills of Fairfax, California, Nischala Devi, draped in purple silk, stands in the doorway of her house—her white, wavy hair falling softly on her shoulders, the breeze mingling with the scent of sandalwood. As we curl up with hot tea on a couch downstairs, her presence is incredibly spacious, as if spending time with me is the most important thing she could possibly be doing at this moment. After talking to her I find myself wondering, what if Patanjali, the great sage who wrote the Yoga Sutras, had been a woman?

The Yoga Sutras of Patanjali are a compilation of 196 aphorisms on the nature of consciousness and liberation. But how do these *sutras* (aphorisms) relate to the life of a modern woman, and how would they be interpreted through a feminine perspective? Yoga teacher Nischala Devi wanted to address that question. So she decided to write a book about it.

"Most of the books are translated by men, from and for a man's consciousness," she says. Considering that most of today's practioners are women, she hopes that her upcoming commentary on the Yoga Sutras, called *The Secret Power of Yoga*, will present these teachings in a new light. "Women can learn yoga through the philosophy and wisdom of the Yoga Sutras. It's the essence of yoga, but people start practicing before they understand what it is they are practicing—and where the practices can lead them."

The last time her views on yoga philosophy were put into writing it created a stir in the yoga community. She was interviewed in 2002 for an article in *Yoga Journal* about her perspective on the male-centric yoga texts, particularly as it related to the Bhagavad Gita, which unfolds as a battlefield dialogue between the warrior prince Arjuna and Lord Krishna. Nischala Devi expressed the need for a more compassionate, heart-centered approach to spiritual practice that honors the emotions, rather than overriding or controlling them. Her version of the story would unfold in a fertile field of love and compassion, rather than on a battlefield. Letters poured in to the editors from women and men alike, some commending her and some outraged at her boldness in questioning these ancient texts.

Stepping out of the mainstream is not new for Nischala Devi. She left a career as a physician's assistant in the 1960s to follow her spiritual path and eventually became a monk. While living in the Satchidananda ashram in Virginia, her pioneering spirit led her to integrate Western medicine and yoga. In 1982, she met two men who independently asked her to help develop health programs. With Michael Lerner she developed the award-winning Commonweal Cancer Help Program, which offers yoga retreats for people with cancer; with Dr. Dean Ornish she created the yoga component of his program for reversing heart disease. She now offers Yoga of the Heart, a training for yoga teachers and health professionals that enables them to work safely and effectively with cardiac and cancer patients. Her book *The Healing Path of Yoga* integrates these teachings. She writes, "Yoga is not a *treatment*, it is a *consciousness* that allows health, balance, and joy to be our companions throughout our entire life's journey."

Nischala's reinterpretation of the Yoga Sutras is evident in her version of one of the most commonly quoted sutras, *yogas citta-vrtti-nirodhah* (1:2), often translated as "yoga is the control of the mental modifications of the mind." Nischala observes, "All the scriptures talk about the light at the center of the heart as *chitta*, and then somehow *chitta* was translated into *mind* and *mental modifications*." Nischala Devi reinterprets this phrase using the metaphor of the ocean as universal consciousness: "Yoga is the uniting of consciousness in

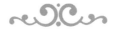

the heart," and "*Chit* is universal consciousness. It also means 'unlimited knowledge.' Everything you can imagine and beyond is in that."

She uses the image of a bottle to represent the individual:

When I am ready to incarnate, my body takes a form. Let's say it takes the form of a water bottle, and someone else incarnates with a body that takes the shape of a wine bottle. If we both incarnate at the same time, we would both walk down to the ocean of consciousness, *chit*, and fill up our newly formed containers. Mine might be short and wide and theirs long and thin, but we both are there to fill up with this sacred consciousness. We then identify with that individual consciousness, or *chitta*, and from the *chitta*, thoughts and feelings are projected. The bottles may appear to be different, but what's inside is never changed. It is always the same. When it's time for me to leave this plane, I take the container, in this case a water bottle, and pour the *chitta* back into the *chit*. It doesn't stay separate even a micro-millimeter of a second; they unite and become one. Yoga is the identification with what is inside, the bottle is merely the container.

Nischala Devi goes on to explain that the confusion seems to have come through the translation. "Even a couple hundred years ago there was no word for mind, or thoughts. Everything came from the heart—thoughts came from the heart, feelings came from the heart." Nischala Devi feels that in our culture, we have separated the mind and the feelings and that this has been reflected in the separation of the male and the female. "In general, women tend to be more feeling and men tend to be more thinking, so the polarity comes in, but really, we all need to think *and* feel, we need to have both sides. Consciousness is in the heart. It can't be touched through control and harsh methods—the heart doesn't respond to that—it responds to kindness and openness and love . . . and it's all in there. Yoga brings us back into the heart, by gathering the consciousness from the body, mind, and emotions and returning it back to the heart. When we have reunited, we are said to be in yoga."

Nischala Devi's roots in the yoga tradition give her a unique vantage point from which to offer a novel perspective on the philosophy and wisdom of yoga. She lived at the ashram of the yoga master Swami Satchidananda for more than eighteen years, where she received his direct guidance and training. She first met him in San Francisco, in 1972. She remembers walking into the hall where he sat. "All the yoga masters, many from India, were sitting up on stage: Yogi Bhajan, Swami Kriyananda, Vishnu Devananda, a Zen teacher, and many others. They gave talks and spoke about their spiritual paths," she says. "There was a glow around Swami Satchidananda. He was emanating light." What resonated with Nischala Devi was his focus on joy. "I really wasn't interested in my spiritual journey being austere or intense; I knew that my true nature was joy." This heart-centered approach to teaching is what draws many students to her retreats, workshops, and trainings around the world today. In her classes there is always laughter, tears, and deep connection.

Satchidananda's teacher, Swami Sivananda, who founded the Divine Light Society in Rishikesh, was a pioneer in his own right. Sivananda was the first teacher Nischala Devi ever heard of who initiated women into the holy order of *sanyas* (monastic tradition), for which he was strongly criticized. She appreciated this movement within the Sivananda lineage towards including women, and the fact that, on the surface at least, gender wasn't an issue. The men washed the dishes and cleaned the toilets; they did everything the women did. The only difference? Swami Satchidananda rarely let the men serve special visiting guests from India who weren't used to being served by men. "It was a cultural issue, but otherwise the women did *puja* (ritual offerings), the women did initiations, it was very equal in that sense. He was very open for an Indian teacher. That's one of the reasons I stayed for as long as I did."

At the Satchidananda ashram, everyone contributed to the community with some form of work; Nischala Devi's was teaching, which led her around the world, teaching in Belgium, Russia, Switzerland, Hungary, Germany, Canada, Costa Rica, and India. As she traveled, her worldview broadened, which influenced and evolved her teaching in a way that eventually led her beyond the traditional ways of the ashram. She found herself particularly challenged by the interpretation of some of the scriptures. When the ashram published a translation of the Yoga Sutras, Nischala Devi sought to have some of the words changed. "Especially *saucha*, which was translated as purity, but was described as 'disgust for one's body and relations with other bodies,'" Nischala Devi says. "I feel as a woman that can't be true. You change a baby's diaper, but you're not disgusted by it. You just change it. You love the baby, so that's just part of the baby. As a woman, I can't translate this as 'disgust for one's own body and for others' bodies.' It's not something that women will tolerate." When she insisted on having the language changed, they told her they couldn't because that was the literal translation from Sanskrit. "I didn't realize at the time that Sanskrit isn't a literal language, but a vibrational language," she says.

When she started teaching Peacock Pose—which is done lying on the belly with the arms tucked under the stomach—Nischala Devi realized that the center of gravity is different in a woman, the breasts have to be considered, and it isn't appropriate to put that much pressure on a woman's belly. "I was teaching the Peacock Pose and I said, wait a minute, women aren't peacocks, they're peahens! A peahen looks totally different from a peacock. I started to question. Well, that's death to a person that's in a tradition. If you start to question too much, you have to leave. Traditions aren't built up over thousands of years because they've been questioned."

Nischala Devi left the ashram in 1991. Although she maintained her commitment to the spirit of her monastic vows—to know herself, to serve and love all—she was changing and seeing things differently. While she contemplated this decision, one of her brother monks said to her, "If there's a large oak tree, when the acorns drop they can't root. They have to fall far enough from the tree to be able to take root within themselves; if they are too close to the tree, they cannot grow." It was time for her to go. "Having been given a great deal of wisdom, it was time to find my own truth and my own way," Nischala Devi says.

It was Indra Devi, known as the mother of modern yoga, who came to midwife her through the transition. Indra Devi had heard that Nischala Devi was leaving the ashram, and knew that Nischala needed guidance. "In a very loving way, she helped me," says Nischala Devi. "It was a difficult time. She gave me the confidence to trust that everything would be as it should be." Indra Devi came to Nischala Devi at the ashram and stayed for two days. "She was giving me words of wisdom, guiding me in the details of what to do, when to leave, with support and love. I realized then that this path doesn't have to be so hard, it can be soft and light."

Today, Nischala Devi shines light on the yoga path by using positive language in her translation of the Yoga Sutras in her classes and workshops. "I changed a lot of the language that was blaming and the 'finger shaking,' as I call it, and focused instead on the fact that we have a compassionate power within us. Most of us are raised on blame and that is where we are most comfortable. Who are we when we see ourselves as divine beings? How are we different when we live our lives from that place?"

In her translation of the Yoga Sutras, she uses words with less emotional charge, such as in her interpretation of *yogas citta-vrtti-nirodhah*. "'Instead of struggling to gain control over the mind and thoughts, make friends with and unite it back into its home at the heart.' The fear of not being able to control something as powerful as the mind is such a trigger. But if you have a yearning for unity and freedom it's very different. It often is as simple as changing the words that alters the meaning and the intensity of the emotion." Nischala Devi's initial orientation to the sutras was intellectual because that's what she learned from her teachers. "I'm having to rework everything. I'm having to take the intellectual understanding and retranslate it from my intuition." She feels that all women have this natural intuition, but tend to rely on outside forces for information and don't develop it. "We all have it, a sense of knowing that we are the one in our essence—men have it, women have it. I think it's more apparent to us as women, but we often don't receive recognition for it. Through embracing our divine nature, this knowing is brought to the forefront of everything we say and do."

Nischala Devi believes there are two parts to every tradition. "There's the kernel of the teachings and all the stories around the teachings," she says. "I go back to the kernel, to get the truth out of it, and that is not held by either sex. The word in Hindi for 'translation' means to 'tell the story in a different way.' So when we talk about tradition, we realize that Master Sivananda broke with tradition, in a large way. By bringing women into the monastic tradition, he made a radical change in the ashram by allowing both men and women to live there. We have to break with tradition too, but still keep the roots. It's O.K. to trim the tree, but you can't destroy the roots. Take the kernel and the essence."

For over thirty years, NISCHALA DEVI has been a highly respected and loved international speaker, teacher, and healer. She spent over eighteen years as a monk receiving direct guidance and teachings from Sri Swami Satchidananda; developed the yoga portion of *The Dean Ornish Program for Reversing Heart Disease*; and cofounded the award-winning *Commonweal Cancer Help Program*. She is author of *The Healing Path of Yoga* and creator of Yoga of the Heart, a training and certification program for yoga teachers and health professionals, designed to adapt yoga practices for cardiac patients. Her latest book is *The Secret Power of Yoga: A Woman's Guide to Bringing a Female Perspective to the Yoga Sutras* (Harmony/Random House, 2007).

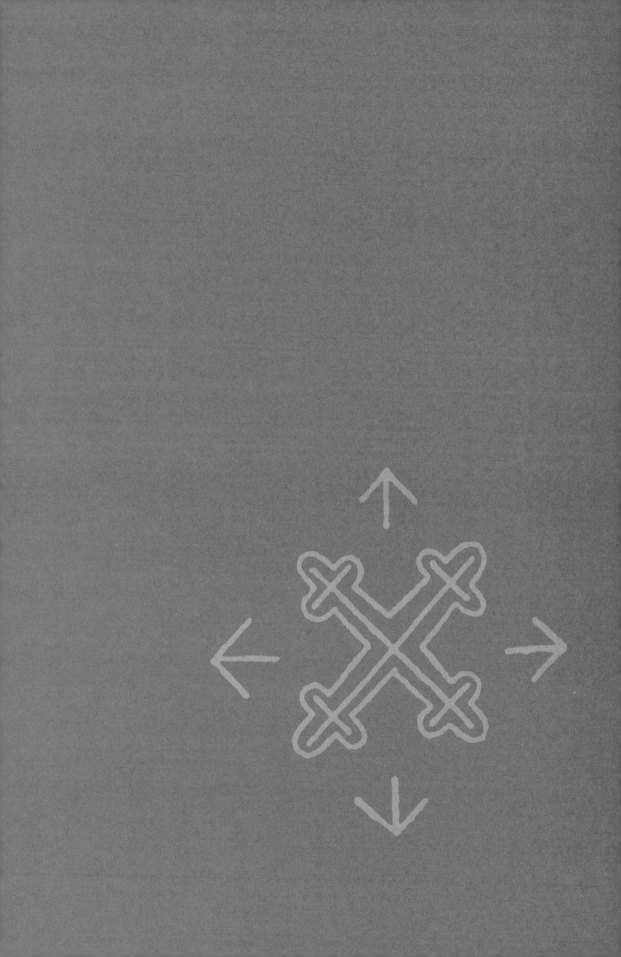

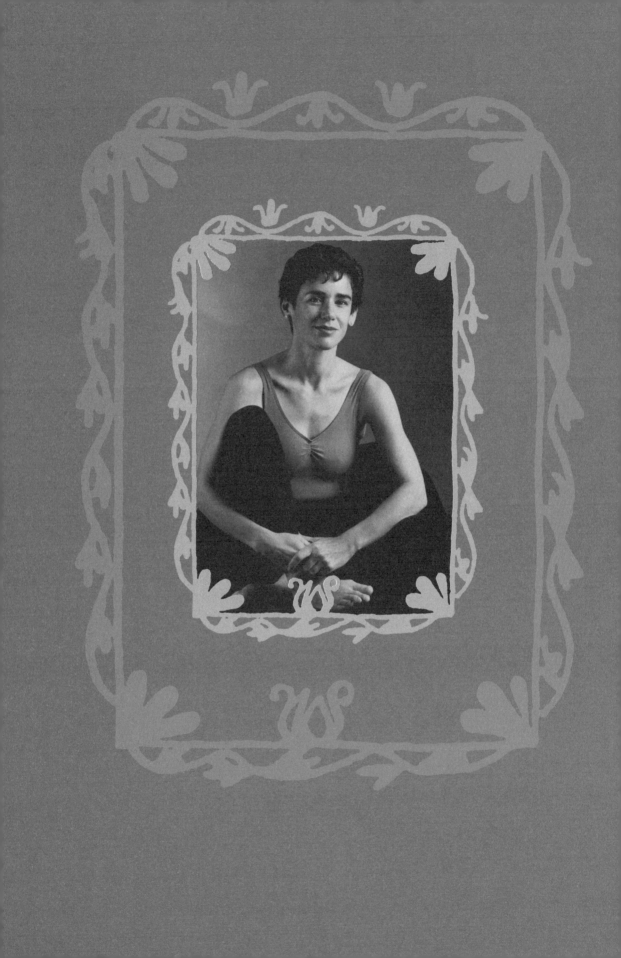

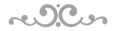

DONNA FARHI

How can we embrace who we are,
where we are, as women in our bodies?

When Donna Farhi was in high school, she took a yoga class as an elective. Through slowing down her breathing, moving through the yoga postures, and focusing her mind, she connected to a part of herself that was safe and content, unaffected by the outer turbulence going on in her life at that time. She started practicing daily and eventually became a sought-after yoga teacher herself. But since that time, Donna says she sees a disturbing trend in the way yoga is practiced. In response to this, she has focused her energy on building a bridge between the physical practice of yoga, which has become so popular, and its spiritual roots.

"The practice of yoga now is being used to create a very strong, explicit identification with the body," says Donna. "That is a 180-degree contradiction to the central tenet of the traditional philosophical underpinning of the practice, which says that we are *more* than our body and that we should identify with not the body itself, but this magnificent force that is animating it." The focus on the physical aspects of yoga practice saddens Donna. "In some sense," she says, "yoga is becoming the practice of a sophisticated form of calisthenics. It has become a part of the pathology of the culture and it's feeding into that pathology." Through her books, workshops, trainings, and retreats around the world, Donna encourages students and teachers alike to rediscover the spiritual essence of yoga, which often gets lost in pursuit of the physical pose. With a depth of knowledge in anatomy, physiology, and the philosophy and psychology of yoga, Donna integrates breathing, movement, and inner inquiry for a practice that teaches not only how to do triangle pose, but how to live an embodied spiritual life.

Donna's teaching reflects her own life experience. During a time of emotional upheaval, Donna and her family moved to New Zealand from the United States when she was ten. She found it challenging to adapt to her new environment and felt she never quite fit in with her high school peers. Overall, she was confused and depressed. She started practicing yoga at the age of sixteen—the same time that she was unwittingly entering a period of anorexia.

Although Donna had discovered a sanctuary of peace and calm through yoga, she continued to struggle with anorexia. It wasn't until she was about eighteen that she realized she had an eating disorder, and although she still didn't know how to deal with it, she knew she had a huge conflict around the need to nourish herself. Based on her experience, she believes that anorexia and other eating disorders are a misdirected spiritual impulse. "When I look at what it was I was seeking, it was the experience of transcendence from a very painful experience of being embodied, because when you're embodied, of course, you feel. And when you have a weighty body, you have a body of substance, then you have a definite feeling." She found that without the weight of food in her body, it was possible to enter an expanded state of consciousness, where there was a sense of being outside the body entirely. Donna realized later that she was truly seeking to discover this transcendent self, but in this misguided effort, she was physically disappearing.

Soon after she discovered yoga, Donna's interest in movement drew her to study dance. Dance provided an experience similar to what she found in yoga: connecting to something larger than herself and giving her a way to express that connection through her body. She became technically proficient, but over time it started to feel mechanical and empty. She lost interest and turned back to yoga.

By the age of nineteen, Donna had moved back to the United States, settling in San Francisco, where she studied Iyengar-style yoga while earning a degree from San Francisco State University. Graduating summa cum laude, her major combined studies in interdisciplinary sciences, religion, and technical writing. Her conflict around eating continued until she was twenty-three, when she met yoga teacher Judith Hanson Lasater, who, Donna says, felt comfortable in her body. "Here was this woman who had a lovely, curvaceous woman's body," Donna says. Up until then she'd only known dance teachers who were emaciated, with no hips or breasts—a body type often held up as the ultimate in femininity. The healthy image Lasater presented helped Donna gain acceptance of her own body. Eventually her conflict around eating completely fell away, which she credits to insights she had in her yoga practice as well as the healing power of her husband's love.

Pursuing her interest in yoga, Donna went to India to study with BKS Iyengar, and then to London to study with Kofi Busia. She also studied with Dona Holleman in Europe. Her training focused on the external form of the poses and was physically challenging. Over time, as she developed her practice and started teaching, she realized she was repeating the experience she had with dance: identifying with the body. Through formal yogic breathing exercises and intensive *asana* (postures), Donna found she was "stepping in the same puddles over and over again," in her work, relationships, and yoga practice. She constantly injured herself. Instead of the sanctuary it had once been, her yoga practice became mechanical and disconnected. She felt the need to find a different way.

In her search, Donna traveled to Greece to study with Angela Farmer, who opened her to the possibilities of a freer, more organic way of practicing. In contrast to how the Iyengar method was taught, Angela encouraged working with ease rather than effort. In the process of practicing in this new way, Donna unearthed old traumas. As her skeletons came out of the closet, she realized she had been using her old controlled practices to unconsciously suppress her fears. She migrated away from both Iyengar's and Farmer's philosophies, feeling one had too much structure and the other too much process. She realized that for her, the true path was the one into her own heart. Discarding techniques and practices, she concluded that only practices that directly focused on opening and nourishing the heart would yield the great results she sought.

Donna began to evolve her own style of teaching, integrating structure and spontaneity—a risk at a time when there wasn't a lot of interest in a practice that wasn't based exclusively on alignment and form. She had very few students at first. Now, she sees a groundswell of students who have taken the physical practice to the limit. "They've done the thirty-minute headstand, the five-minute handstand, and the 108 backbends. These students are now asking, 'Is this all there is?' It leaves them empty." Her students are now interested in learning the essence of the practice and discovering ways to embody it. "You may discover yourself through those rigid forms, but the forms in and of themselves are empty. It's what animates those forms that is to be connected to."

At her women's retreats, Donna focuses on encouraging women to cultivate acceptance not as they wish they could be at some future time, but as they truly are at this moment. "Women wouldn't in a million years treat their best friend the way they treat themselves. And yet on a daily basis there's this terrible judgment or internal critic that's refusing to acknowledge who they are. It's constantly an act of refusing." At these retreats, she incorporates activities that bring about an embracing of the body. Recently, she led students in body casting, where women choose a part of their body that they are most unhappy with and cover it in plaster. When the plaster dries, they can see from a new perspective the parts they have previously rejected. "One hundred percent of the time, the women take [the cast] off and look and say, 'Oh my God, I have a beautiful bottom, I have beautiful thighs. How could I ever have thought this about my body?'"

Donna also emphasizes the importance of creating a sacred and safe space for yoga practice. She does this primarily by creating an atmosphere of self-responsibility: she tells her students not to believe anything she tells them and to question everything based on their own experience. And then she tells them to let her know if they arrive at some different answers so she can share that information with others. This gives students room to have their own experiences and to voice them without feeling as though they are being disrespectful or that they would be criticized for challenging her perception. "When you're in inquiry with an attitude of curiosity and an attitude of delight for the process, you take the fear away."

This emphasis on sacred and safe space extends to the ethical issues of the student-teacher relationship, a topic that has spawned numerous conversations at conferences across the country. "The longer I teach, the more I realize what an immense responsibility I hold." She feels that if a teacher is aware of the depth to which the practice can take a student and understands how this practice of transformation makes a student vulnerable, the teacher would never want to violate that process. In her teacher trainings, Donna emphasizes the importance of teachers looking outside of their community of students as much as possible to meet their social, emotional, intellectual, and sexual needs. She says, "Not that we hide anything from the students, but the student is not there to meet my needs, ever. I am there to meet theirs. I don't walk into the room needing reassurance, or needing the students to stroke my ego, or needing the students to find me attractive or strong or whatever. I need to be there as a neutral vessel through which these students are going to have an experience of transformation."

Donna has had long correspondences and dialogues with women who have been in abusive relationships with their male teachers, and she's familiar with the impact these transgressions can have on a student. She advises women who may have a history of seeking their self-worth through a man to seek out a female teacher. She sees that a central issue for these women is a lack of belief in themselves as more than just a body.

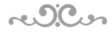

Donna feels strongly that neither the students' nor the teachers' lack of wholeness will be addressed by having an affair. "The problem for the woman is that she doesn't see herself. She doesn't see how special, wonderful, and magnificent she is and that's why she thinks she needs to find someone outside of herself who is going to be like the talent scout that comes to town and discovers her. No, she has to discover herself. Whether it's with her teacher or a relationship with anyone, it's always going to be seeking this outside eye that's going to witness her true self."

One of the things that Donna is exploring as a teacher, with both her male and female students, is the acceptance that all parts of the self need to come out onto the mat. She also sees the importance of a healthy acceptance of our sexual and sensual parts. "When we don't allow that energy to come through us in a whole and natural way, then it comes out in very perverse, destructive ways. You can't say 'I'll allow every part of the self to express itself except this' because it's a big one, it's a hugely powerful energy. If we allow and we create a safe container around them for ourselves and others, we don't misuse these energies."

Donna describes herself as a global citizen, having gone back and forth all her life between the United States and New Zealand, with their different values. Now, while at home on her thirty acres in the countryside of North Canterbury on the South Island of New Zealand, she gets up at dawn to feed her horses, clean out the paddock, and attend to the land. In contrast, when she is touring, Donna commutes across oceans to work, teaching in Europe, the U.S., and Canada. Living close to nature while on her farm in New Zealand helps her return to balance. "I think the connection with nature for me has to do with recalibrating myself to a primordial rhythm. Most of us are out of sync with that rhythm; we're going too fast for too long. So to be in sync with that rhythm can mean very basic things, such as I get up at dawn because the sun's getting up. I go to sleep because I'm tired."

An integral part of Donna's practice today is caring for her horses. "They demand such a depth of observation . . . they can't speak to us in our language, but they do speak through their body language, through very subtle things that they do or don't do—a change in the look in their eyes can indicate something. It requires of me a level of focus and concentration that I haven't even experienced in the most intensive meditation retreat." Attuning to this subtlety has humbled Donna. "I find my horses are my strongest and most powerful teachers. They have an amazing ability to discover what is stuck in you and once they discover what is stuck in you they aren't going to budge until you change— not until they change, until *you* change." Now, she hopes to share what excites her on a

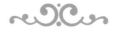

deep level with others. "Fifteen years ago it might have been doing 108 backbends, but that's not true now for me anymore. It's not what excites me or moves my heart. What really moves my heart is seeing people change on a really deep, deep level, coming to love themselves and coming to be more loving and trusting with others."

DONNA FARHI has been practicing yoga for thirty years and teaching since 1982. She is one of the most sought-after guest teachers in the world, leading intensives and teacher-training programs internationally. Donna is best known for her unique ability to help students and teachers embody their spiritual practice. Her work focuses on the refinement of natural and universal movement principles that underlie all yoga practice. Donna has been the asana columnist for both *Yoga Journal* and *Yoga International* magazines, and has been profiled in three separate publications on outstanding contemporary teachers of our time. Donna is the author of *The Breathing Book, Yoga Mind, Body & Spirit: A Return to Wholeness,* and *Bringing Yoga to Life: The Everyday Practice of Enlightened Living.* Born in America, Donna now resides in Christchurch, New Zealand, where she pursues her passionate love of horses.

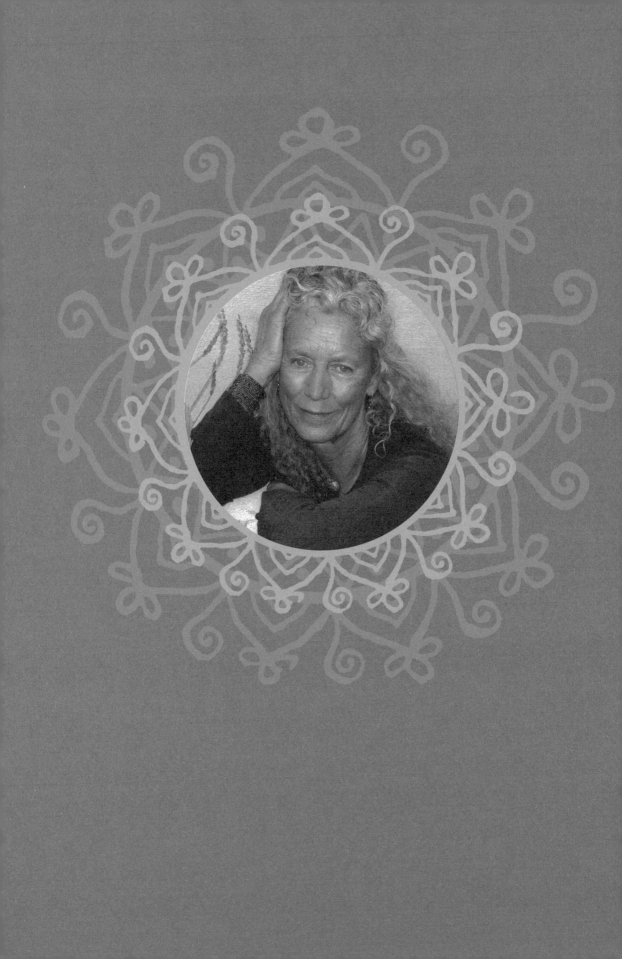

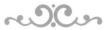

ANGELA FARMER

We cannot strive towards
something that we already are.

One night, after a long quest looking for a spiritual teacher that culminated in Dharamsala, India, Angela Farmer went out into the night and looked out over the Himalayan peaks and the plains below. "The Tibetans were in the nearby temples playing their long horns that sent a haunting sound echoing around the hills, punctuated with the occasional crash of cymbals. It felt as if the whole earth was opening up!" At that moment she heard a voice say, "The teacher is within."

With this clear insight, she let go of her search for guidance and began a new journey. Near Orissa, in the south of India, she came across a temple by the sea. Carved into the stone temple were sensual, female figures with bare breasts and round bellies, dancing and playing the flute with ecstatic smiles on their faces: blissful yoginis. The image that Angela had cherished for the previous ten years, of the emaciated yogi sitting in a cave meditating, instantly dissolved. "It was like a lightning bolt through my body," she says. She realized that it was acceptable to practice yoga in a feminine way. A mirror of her own potent internal female energy, these voluptuous, flowing Hindu goddesses served as her initiation into the feminine. Years later, she and her partner Victor Van Kooten began teaching together and called their approach "yoga from the inside out." It has drawn both men and women seeking an alternative to the masculine, goal-oriented style.

Returning home to her own feminine nature, Angela's yoga practice began to change as she started listening to herself more. "My body wanted to move, it didn't want to be stuck in a rigid pose," she says. As Angela unraveled her own pains and opened to her emotions, she cried an "ocean of tears." For the first time in many years, her menstrual cycle, which had stopped due to the intensive physical practices, returned. She began to uncover a whole new part of herself as well as her yoga. "The taste of undoing was so much more delicious than the taste of doing," Angela says.

"I began to slowly understand that the intellect is very fast . . . it judges very quickly and then tries to fix. But the body is slower, it has a totally different intelligence, which comes about through instinct and feelings and old, old understandings," she says. For Angela, the breath, the belly, and the back body are essential elements of a yoga practice. She encourages students to gently open these neglected parts of themselves with awareness, to fill them with breath, give them direction through movement, and thus discover a practice that can be both healing and empowering. "Awakening awareness of the perineum and the possibility of reconnecting to the earth through envisioned roots brings about a deep sense of peace and grounding so often lacking in our goal-oriented and speeded-up lifestyle."

Angela has spent much of her life exploring how to remap the internal energy network and heal the body. When she was a teenager, she had invasive surgery that left her with diminished nerve control. To treat a circulation problem they feared would lead to gangrene, doctors cut and removed sympathetic nerves that connected her spinal cord to her extremities in the cervical and lumbar areas, leaving scar tissue, metal clips, and pain. After the surgery, she lost a great deal of sensation, her hands and feet couldn't sweat anymore, and her energy was vastly depleted. In response, she developed a specific practice of directing energy through her body, guiding it to the extremities to bring life back to her hands and feet.

"Energy follows imagery," Angela says. This energy (*prana*) is now a central focus of her teaching. Through imagery, fluid movement, and conscious breathing, she guides students to explore this power that animates the body. The perineum becomes a flower, opening and closing, a gathering point of energy. Feet grow roots down into the earth, shoulder blades expand into wings, inner rivers course along spiral pathways. Angela sees the yoga postures (*asanas*) as having evolved out of this process of connecting with and activating the subtle body. She asks, "Where are our stuck places?" The "stuck

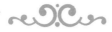

places" are those parts where feeling is avoided, is numb entirely, or is rejected outright. Angela invites students to delve into these areas and to open a dialogue with them. "We do a lot of yoga postures, but are we really going into the unknown?" Angela asks. A belly full of scar tissue, old injuries, and chronic pain have inspired Angela to become intimate with those parts of herself. She encourages others to do the same. "The places where you have particular issues, particular fears or pains or dark sides, that's where the treasure lies." Her work is in helping people find the courage to uncover these obscured areas, to bring back their embodied sense of self-empowerment, and in the process discover "that they are full of potency, beauty, love, and everything they need."

Of her early experience with traditional yoga training, Angela says, "I had been very well trained to judge what was correct and what was incorrect. There was this high expectation of perfection, striving, judging oneself . . . one's body was never good enough." She found that for most students, the body rarely fit into the shape of the poses the way it was expected to. "Periodically it would and you'd have a flash and it would be fantastic. The energy would be roaring through you." But then it was gone. There was always the underlying pain and struggle, the vulnerable places in the body that had been injured or traumatized. She felt that there was no room for them to emerge and that these traumas had to hide away inside. "I'd built an armor around them and managed to do the poses keeping them nicely locked inside."

Angela knows from her own experience how deeply some of these traumas are buried in the body. While teaching a women's intensive at Kripalu Center for Yoga & Health in Lenox, Massachusetts, she had some bodywork from a craniosacral therapist. The session unearthed an experience that led to an injury when she was eight years old. In the next session, Angela went back to the trauma of being sexually abused at the age of ten months.

"I thought I'd never get off of the table. I thought, 'How could anyone do such a horrible thing to a child?'" The therapist showed her the way of compassion, telling her that people do what has been done to them. After the session, Angela went straight back to teaching her workshop. "I saw these women in a whole new light," she says. She asked how many had been sexually abused. When two-thirds of the hands went up, tears started to flow. At a recent *Yoga Journal* conference, she taught a workshop specifically addressing this issue.

With her long, lean limbs, flowing gray hair, and dangling earrings, Angela embodies what she teaches. There is a catlike suppleness to her gait, and she artfully adapts her teaching to flow with whatever arises. On September 11, 2001, she was teaching her annual ten-day women's retreat at Harbin Hot Springs in California, when the airplanes crashed into the World Trade Center. When someone informed the group of the tragic news, the energy started to escalate and fear filled the room. Angela gathered the women together in a circle, grounding and focusing their attention to hold a sacred space in the middle of the chaos. Later, one woman arrived in the aftermath of being stuck in transit for two days amongst the confusion. Again, when the group's questions started creating an atmosphere of anxiety, Angela brought it back into a healing circle. Like the archetypal mother, she wrapped the overwrought woman in a blanket and, along with several other students, rocked her like a baby.

Angela's journey toward this nourishing and feminine approach evolved over a period of many years. "When I was young, God lived in the sky and men were on pedestals," Angela says. As a child, she was deeply religious, and all of the great saints and teachers she admired were male. Having no female image to mirror her own divine nature, she developed a sense of inadequacy as a woman. This drove her to negate what she saw as feminine. Growing up with two brothers further reinforced this belief. "In my deep unconscious I grew up thinking that men were better than women because they get everything, and the women take care of the men back home and then they have children and take care of *them*." Her brothers went to nice schools with beautiful facilities, laboratories, soccer, tennis, and multiple career opportunities. Angela was expected to stay home and help. She was told to be quiet and not express her opinion. As was true for most women before the feminist movement exploded in the 1960s, her life choices were limited to being a wife and mother, a nurse, a teacher, or a secretary. She yearned for something more.

Angela decided to become a schoolteacher because it offered her an opportunity to travel. While teaching in England in 1967 when she was twenty-eight, she had her first yoga class, with a woman named Diana Clifton. After six months, her teacher introduced her to BKS Iyengar, now one of the most well-known and respected yoga teachers in the world. Drawn to his methods and expertise, she studied with him for more than ten years. "I loved the challenge of yoga as I learned it. Especially in the beginning, it appealed to my more athletic side." In 1975, Angela went to India to study with Iyengar for three months. At that time, he didn't have an institute, just a small room in a house. "It was exciting . . . his way of teaching was to bash you down so you felt totally nothing, that

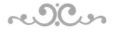

everything you did was totally wrong and you would come out totally desperate. You'd go back the next day and he'd build you up and you'd feel great and the next day he'd bash you down again. It's not an easy way to learn, but he was very interested in and passionate about the process. I felt that underneath it all he had a good heart and was a good man."

Angela gradually recognized that this method of teaching was based on fear. "I didn't realize at the time because I had so much deep fear inside me, hidden away in the cells and pulling into the bone. So for me to follow a fear-based teacher or teaching was just a continuation. It was challenging me further and further into the warrior phase." Angela kept practicing harder and harder, often before and after class. She recalls one day coming out of a backbend and dropping into a deep sleep, exhausted. "I didn't feel fluid. Somewhere inside I knew I had to leave this approach. But at the same time, I had this feeling that if I just left it without really understanding why, there would be that little voice inside me saying 'You chickened out. It was too hard, too painful for you . . . coward!'" So she continued until it became very clear that this was not creating the changes she needed. "Being a warrior, I wasn't going to be defeated."

The transition in Angela's teaching style from the traditional Iyengar method, with its emphasis on alignment, form, and straight lines to one of inner exploration where the body moves in arcs and spirals, was not easy. Although she was one of the few who held an advanced teaching certificate from Iyengar, students were told that they could no longer study with Angela or her partner Victor Van Kooten and simultaneously expect to pursue their studies with the Iyengar method. Both Angela's and Victor's class attendance dropped from sixty students to six. "It was like being excommunicated," she says.

Some have questioned whether her organic way of practicing is really yoga. In her class, one person may be rolling over a ball, while another is in downward-facing dog with one leg shaking out to the side—bodies undulating within the pose, as each individual explores and evolves the posture to fit their own needs. However, it's clear that others respond to her innovative approach. Today, students from all yoga traditions flock to the workshops she and Victor teach around the world, both independently and together, including their "Teacher Untraining." Donna Farhi, Rama Jyoti Vernon, Barbara Benagh, and many other prominent female teachers acknowledge that Angela was their role model. Empowering them through her living example, Angela's pioneering

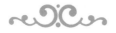

path paved the way for them to discover their own personal relationship to the practice of yoga, staying true to themselves in their practice and in their teaching. "I feel we really need to find it within ourselves. We need to *refind* the truth within ourselves."

———————

Angela Farmer has been teaching yoga for over thirty-five years. After traveling to India to study with BKS Iyengar, she began exploring her own approach to yoga. In 1984, she and Victor Van Kooten joined their teachings to develop a unique style that focuses on the feminine as a way to find peace and compassion. Angela has produced two videos, *The Feminine Unfolding* and *A Flow Class with Angela*.

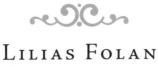

LILIAS FOLAN

Whether the outer shell is male or female,
the inner is without gender. I just happen to
have a female outer shell this lifetime.
I enjoy being in a female body, but eventually
I'm going to even let that go.

*I*n the early 1960s, Lilias Folan lived in a white clapboard house in Darien, Connecticut, with her husband, two children, and two golden retrievers. It was the picture-perfect life. But she was miserable. At twenty-eight, she didn't even know how to label her experience. She went to her doctor complaining of back pain and fatigue. "I was carrying a fairly large gloom cloud, one that was from the psychological and emotional aspects of my being. But there was also a deep sense of not knowing a higher power, the light, God, whatever one wanted to call it. I felt bereft. It took many years to understand that and how to return to the heart."

Now, at the age of sixty-seven, Lilias Folan—often called "The First Lady of Yoga" because she introduced millions of Americans to yoga with her PBS television series *Lilias! Yoga and You*—continues to develop her practice and helps others to do the same. Lilias's TV series ran from 1972 to 1985, and featured a young Lilias in long braid and leotard, translating the teachings of yoga into terms that people of all ages, shapes, and sizes could understand. Today, with short hair and loose-fitting clothing, she is turning her attention to the growing number of students aged fifty and older who attend her workshops across the country. Lilias is inspired by these students, who come seeking a practice that's comfortable for their aging bodies, but also with a deep yearning for peace and contentment and for living in the present moment. "There is an energy that is exchanged now that has to do with the spirit. I really see that we can get right down to it. I don't have to beat around the bush."

Like many of her students, an underlying desire for happiness originally drew her to yoga. With a recommendation from her doctor to start a program of physical exercise, Lilias intuitively found her way to a yoga class at the local YWCA. Her practice was inspired by one of the few accessible books on yoga at the time, *Yoga, Youth and Reincarnation* by Jess Stearn. As she read the book, Lilias recognized that Stearn was addressing the lesser-known parts of her self: the mental, emotional, and spiritual. It was a window to the inside, and she wanted to open it wider. "I was hurting physically, but mentally there was a lot of healing that needed to happen. As with many cases, discomfort, mental anguish, and physical pain help people to change. It can be a very compassionate teacher."

Fortunately for Lilias, she didn't have to run off to India to pursue her interest in yoga. "India was coming to New York," she says. It was an exciting time and she met many of the teachers who came to the United States from India, planting the seeds of yoga in American soil. Lilias studied with Swamis Vishnu Devananda and Satchidananda of the Sivananda lineage, and eventually found solace in the ashram of the Divine Light Society. Her Christian roots gave her a familiarity and a sense of safety at the ashram, which was only an hour's drive from her home in Connecticut. "I fell in love with all the ritual, the beauty of the altar, and the candles." The president of the Divine Light Society, Swami Chidananda, became her primary teacher.

When yoga master Swami Muktananda, founder of Siddha yoga, who was known for his ability to transmit *shakti* (energy), came through New York City in the 1980s, Swami Chidananda encouraged Lilias to go see him. "I went up with everyone else to get a few words. . . . He said, 'You are the real thing, and you must start to teach meditation.' Well, I was shocked. I was a little housewife from Darien, Connecticut. Whoa!"

As Lilias fell passionately in love with yoga, through the changes she saw in her body and in her being, it became difficult for her husband and two sons (five and seven at the time) to relate to her experiences. Although her husband loved and supported her, it was confusing for him. "They were really challenging years," Lilias says. At one point she felt called to leave family life altogether. While on a peaceful, early morning boat ride with her husband on Long Island Sound, she felt a deep stirring in her chest, "like a big thumb was pressing from the inside out," accompanied by waves of bliss and a sense of longing. Conflicted about the meaning of this experience, she went to her teacher, Swami Chidananda. Should she leave her family to follow her spiritual path and dedicate her life to God? He acknowledged the experience she had as a call to serve God, but told her that since she had been called *after* her marriage, her spiritual path was within family life—not in an ashram or convent. Although difficult at the time, she now knows that she didn't have to go any further than her own home to learn about love, truth,

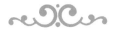

wisdom, and humility. Now with two grown sons, two daughters-in-law, seven grand-children, and a marriage of forty-five years, she has found plenty of opportunity for spiritual growth in her own backyard. The gurus that inspire Lilias on a daily basis today are these intimate family members.

The evolution in Lilias's teaching over the years parallels her own growth. "Forty years ago I was the only kid on the block. Today, I feel a little simpler and clearer about the practice. I'm more accepting of who I am and my spiritual nature; I'm not so embarrassed about it." While her television program focused on the physical postures, today Lilias teaches students to get to know the *sakshin* (witness), this aspect of the self that observes the body, the mind, and the emotions without judgment. Lilias calls this observer "one of my best friends." Meditating and developing this witness consciousness have become essential elements for Lilias in her practice and in her life. After teaching yoga around the world, writing several books, and producing numerous award-winning videos, DVDs, and CDs—even being called the "Julia Child of Yoga" by *Time* magazine—Lilias still has moments of self-doubt. "I'm still struggling with this restless mind, but it's a heck of a lot better than it was thirty years ago."

For the past fifteen years, along with psychologist Marti Glen, she has been co-leading the annual women's retreat at Feathered Pipe Ranch in Montana, where Lilias encourages a sense of self-acceptance. The workshops integrate psychological and spiritual work through yoga, song, dance, and sweat-lodge ceremonies. "It's deep work," Lilias says. Women of all ages return every year, bringing their mothers, daughters, cousins, and sisters, sharing their stories and cultivating this awakened presence. "Different things come up. Humans are all pretty much alike, it just comes out in different ways and sometimes with different forces." She acknowledges that the energy on these retreats is more relaxed and comfortable than if men were there, but she feels the essence of the teachings is beyond gender. "It is something unseen and mystical and I don't know the answer. I call it 'The sacred don't know.'" While Lilias herself enjoys being a woman, she says, "Whether I'm a male or a female, I don't really think about it anymore. The ageless spirit—now *that* interests me."

Lilias's newest book, *Yoga Gets Better with Age*, reflects this focus on spirit. In this book, she takes readers on a journey through the different sheaths that obscure this inner, unchanging light, and the different aspects of our being: the physical, mental, emotional, and spiritual. Written as if she were once again teaching her TV audience in their living rooms in her simple, straightforward way, she guides readers through different layers of themselves, beginning with the physical body. Of her students over the age of fifty she says, "They have to take care and not do every type of yoga that's out there. It will be injurious." Honoring the seasons of life and the need to adapt the practice as we age, she teaches a yin approach to the postures that is cool, calm, and focused, and includes warming up thoroughly. These practices go through the layers and lead to meditation, the key to accessing the inner light.

Her new approach is partially the result of her sense of her own mortality; in turn, she reminds us of our own. "Time is going by and life is swiftly changing. I feel very conscious of this and am very appreciative of having good health at this point. And there are no guarantees about anything." As she's gotten older, she has witnessed friends who've gotten cancer and feel guilty about it, and others who have gone through chemotherapy and handled it with dignity and grace. "This is how I want to be. I'd like to be fairly conscious when I leave this body, I really would." How do we prepare for that moment? "I think it's just dropping into stillness, letting go of the body daily, and contemplating that."

After forty years of practicing yoga and thirty-three years of teaching, how does Lilias avoid burnout? A lifelong learner, she continues to maintain the vitality of her own practice and her teaching by taking classes with other teachers and reading inspirational books. Recently she spent a week with Angela Farmer at Feathered Pipe Ranch. Lilias has also attended a weekend with Eckhart Tolle, accompanied by her husband Bob, who now shares her philosophical and spiritual interests. Bob also practices yoga with her—primarily to improve his golf game.

Lilias is currently fascinated by the *Advaita* (non-dualism) philosophy of Ramana Maharshi, a self-realized saint who taught a method of self-inquiry in which the seeker focuses continuous attention on the "I-thought" to find its source. In the beginning, this requires effort, but eventually something deeper than the ego takes over and the mind dissolves in the heart center. "I feel that this has helped me to simplify things, to meditate on a daily basis, to have a breathing practice on a daily basis, and just to keep my life simple. And continually questioning, who am I? Who am I really? So, that kind of narrows my life down. I don't have to go out so much and find it out there. It's in here. Inside the being, inside the heart, that's where it is."

LILIAS FOLAN is known to many as the "First Lady of Yoga," due to her groundbreaking PBS yoga series *Lilias!* which continues to air on PBS stations today. She began her yoga practice in 1964 and has studied with some of the finest teachers from India, Europe, and the United States, including TKV Desikachar, Angela Farmer, and BKS Iyengar. She is author of *Lilias! Yoga and You; Lilias, Yoga, and Your Life;* and *Lilias! Yoga Gets Better with Age.*

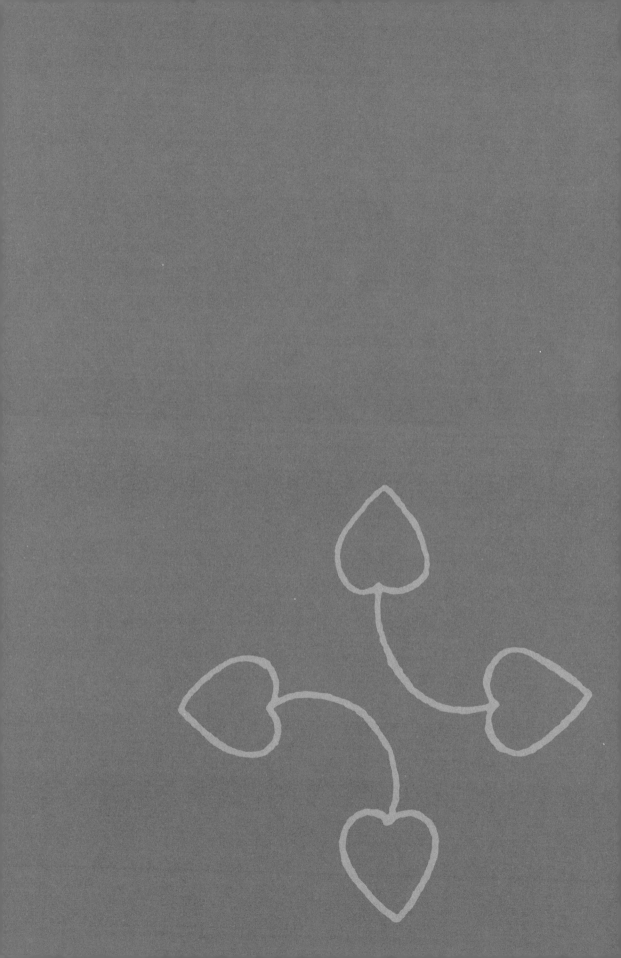

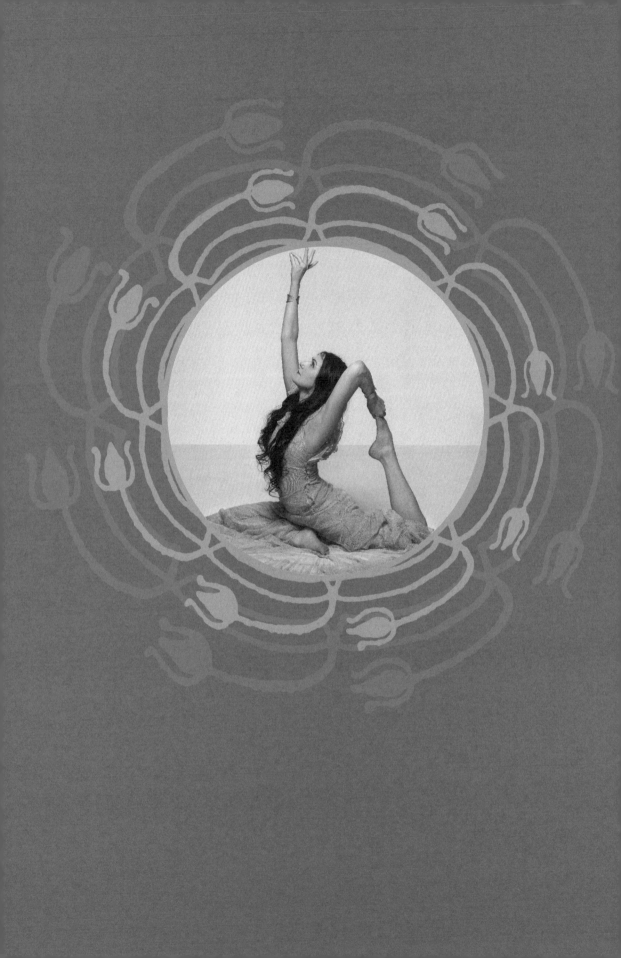

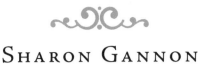

SHARON GANNON

Everything depends on our relationship with
others. How we treat others will
determine how others treat us. How others
treat us will determine how
we see ourselves, and how we see ourselves
will determine who we are.

"All of us in this room are interested in yoga, right?" Sharon Gannon asks the fifty students in this class at a San Francisco yoga conference. She places her clear, direct gaze on the students, making eye contact with one and then another, and another. "But what is yoga interested in?" She pauses to let the question sink in. "Yoga has only one interest, and that is enlightenment. And what is realized in this nirvanic, ecstatic, luminous state? The Oneness of Being; our separate identity is expanded to include the whole, *jivamukti*. *Jiva* is the individual and *mukti* means liberation. Yoga heals the disease of disconnect."

Sharon's yoga is not one of quiet contemplation, and when she opens her mouth, it is on purpose. Hers is an in-your-face spirituality, rooted in the yoga tradition that requires an examination of all your actions and interactions with others. An animal-rights activist and outspoken advocate of ethical veganism, Sharon was nominated "Gutsiest Woman of the Year 1999" by *Jane* magazine. In 2003, her image appeared on a billboard in Times Square behind the New Year's ball, beside a message advocating yoga and vegetarianism as steps towards world peace. She is cocreator of the Jivamukti Yoga method, and codirector of Jivamukti Yoga, one of the largest yoga centers in the world. Although it may be difficult to imagine, this sophisticated, articulate yogini and artist was at one time a bookish librarian "who didn't know her right from her left." What transformed Sharon from an awkward girl into the force she has become today?

A wake-up call. In the aftermath of a traumatic experience when she was twenty-two years old, Sharon weighed only eighty-five pounds and no longer wanted to live. She even attempted suicide. Fortunately, her sister came to her rescue and helped Sharon realize the impact that taking her own life would have on others. It was a turning point. "I realized this was not the way. I needed to pick myself up and give something back to the world." Having hit bottom herself, she felt she had to find a way to help others pull themselves out of their own suffering and unhappiness.

The library where Sharon worked at the time wasn't just any library, it was Seattle's Theosophical Lending Library. With an interest in mysticism nourished by her Catholic upbringing, Sharon was drawn to studying ancient texts and was fascinated by the alchemists. Over the next seven years, she developed a meditation practice and turned to the writings of J. Krishnamurti, Annie Besant, and Charles W. Littlefield, as well as the classical texts on yoga: Patanjali's Yoga Sutras, the Hatha Yoga Pradipika, and the Bhagavad Gita. She began the process of coming into her own strength and power. "Nobody was going to listen to this girl who was afraid of her own shadow. I realized I could be this little bookworm in the library, but it wasn't doing anyone any good." To reconnect with her body, she studied various dance forms, including modern, classical Indian, and ballet; she was graduated from the University of Washington with a degree in dance. Through her training in the performing arts, Sharon learned to express her ideas through movement and music.

Together with her intellectual, artist, and activist friends, Sharon created a magazine, *Patio Table*, produced plays, started a band, organized protest marches, and formed book-study groups. They called themselves Citizens for a Non-Linear Future. Within this group, she was deemed the "spiritual one." During this period, in 1979, she saw *The Animals' Film*, a graphic documentary on the exploitation of animals that she credits for turning her world upside down and putting her firmly on the road of her life's work. "I was trying to find a way to be an effective speaker on the subject of our culture's acceptance of violence and especially the exploitation of animals, nature, and each other." Sharon was struggling to find her voice. "I knew that this voice had to be strong, it had to be correctly informed, but it also had to be kind." She wanted to find a way to apply the spiritual teachings in a very active way "without the anger and blame which seemed to motivate many of my friends."

At that point her only exposure to the practice of yoga postures had been a class she took in 1973 where everyone was "rolling around on the floor," and she hadn't seen much value in it. When Sharon moved to New York in 1983, she wound up working as a waitress at Life Café, a restaurant owned by her future partner, David Life. Sharon suffered from serious back pain, and another waitress, a yoga instructor named Tara Rose, encouraged her to try the practice again. The yoga helped and this time Sharon was hooked. "I began to get at the cause of why I behaved the way I did and why my own life was as it was. I felt it in my body. Our bodies are the storehouse for all the actions we have ever taken." Inspired to learn more and with a desire to share what she was learning, Sharon sought out teachers in New York and beyond. She became certified in the Sivananda style and eventually found her way to India and teachers Sri Brahmananda Saraswati, Swami Nirmalananda, and Sri K. Pattabhi Jois. "Fundamental to the teachings of yoga is the idea of *karma*. It dawned on me that if I could help people make the connection between how we treat others and how we are eventually treated, then I could contribute toward making this world a kinder place."

Today the bookish, introverted girl is nowhere to be seen, but her own journey of transformation has given Sharon insight into what many women experience today. "Most women in our culture don't feel confident." She points to how men are taught that their confidence or power is derived from how many others they can control and how much money they can make by exercising that control. "Women, by our very nature, are reluctant to accept that, so we're kind of lost. Where do we get our confidence? In our sex appeal? In the kind of clothes we're wearing? In the kind of guys we attract?" Like most women, Sharon finds these alternatives superficial and unsatisfying. "When you start to feel the real confidence that comes from yoga, that comes from connecting with that transcendental, eternal self, it is extremely liberating."

While Sharon has no doubt that the practice of yoga has the potential to return us to wholeness, she feels women can often misunderstand the teachings of yoga that stress humility and service. "Because we've been doormats for so long, it's very difficult to know the difference between what it means to be humble and what it means to be humiliated."

Sharon feels that the "indoctrination" of our culture has influenced the way that yoga is being taught in the West. "In most yoga classes, the philosophy of yoga tends to be separate from the physical practice of *asana*. This separation happens because our whole culture separates the body from the mind." Relating the intellect to the masculine and the body to the feminine, she says, "We live in a culture where all things feminine have been relegated to a lesser place."

When the place where Sharon taught lost its lease, her students (her partner David Life among them) encouraged her to find a place to continue to teach. She decided that if she were going to open a yoga center, she didn't want to do it without David and recruited him to teach. Shortly after, in 1986, the duo opened their first Jivamukti Yoga Center in New York, a small studio with purple walls that they quickly outgrew. They moved to a larger space and, since then, Jivamukti has grown and expanded into one of the largest, most popular yoga centers in the world. Sharon and David act as spiritual guides to independently owned Jivamukti Yoga Centers in London, Munich, Toronto, and Detroit; they have also coauthored two books, *Jivamukti Yoga: Practices for Liberating Body & Soul* and *The Art of Yoga*. Jivamukti Yoga classes are dynamic and energetic, infused with philosophy, music, and a purpose-driven spirituality that breathes a modern vitality into the ancient teachings of yoga. Once asked by a television reporter what they taught at Jivamukti, Sharon answered, "Vegetarianism, environmental consciousness, and political activism." In an attempt to steer the interview, the reporter tried again, "What are the physical benefits of yoga?" Sharon's answer: "What could be more physical than what you eat, where you live, and who you live with?"

For Sharon, it all comes back to the primary teachings of yoga, which are the teachings of *karma*. "That everything we're experiencing in our lives is coming from one source—how we've treated others and how we've treated ourselves." This view is woven into her understanding and teaching of the yoga postures. Referring to the Yoga Sutras of Patanjali, the classical teachings on yoga, she says, "*sthira-sukham-asanam* (YSII.46) means that our connection to the earth should be steady and joyful." Sharon translates *asana* as "seat," or our connection to the earth. "Earth means all beings and all things. The Divine manifests in physical form as the Earth: the Divine Feminine." Linking hatha yoga to its roots in the Tantric tradition, which honors the Divine in her female form, Sharon says, "The yogi is a worshipper of the Divine Mother and the Divine Mother is no other than this world and all these beings and everything that appears as 'other.'" According to Sharon, the yoga tradition says that our relationship to the earth—and to all beings— should be mutually beneficial. "It should be based in joy, *sukham*, and it should be steady, *shtira*, meaning under all circumstances, not only if the other is someone that you like or is giving you something you want. It has to be a steady connection at all times."

Sharon emphasizes that as long as we see ourselves as separate from others and perceive our experiences as coming from "out there"—not understanding that our world appears the way it does because of our own projections and past actions—we will suffer. According to yoga philosophy, the negative emotions of how we've treated others and how we've treated ourselves are stored in the energy body as a karmic residue. Sharon describes the physical body of bones, muscles, and blood as the outer manifestation of this internal energy form. She uses the image of branches in winter: When ice freezes on the branches, it takes on the form of the branch. In the same way, the physical body takes on the form of the energy body. "When we practice *asana*, we encounter our resistance to the natural state of wholeness, which is there due to unresolved *karmas*." Sharon feels that if we can help others understand that pain and suffering is not coming from some outside source, "then this whole syndrome of blaming, getting angry, depressed, or sad will be less interesting and we will begin to move in a different direction.

"So, whenever we have an opportunity to relate to someone else, that's an opportunity to clear up our *karmas*." That is why the Jivamukti Yoga method emphasizes what Sharon calls "political activism as spiritual activation." Sharon feels that if she can help people, especially other women, realize that "if we want equality for ourselves as women, and if we want to be honored for our femininity and not be degraded or exploited by it, then we must provide equality, respect, and protection to all other women." Sharon extends this to females of the animal kingdom as well; she encourages women to make conscious choices about what to wear, what to eat, and what to feed their families.

When Sharon made the decision to offer her life in service to the Divine Mother, she looked for a way she could benefit others and somehow not contribute to the ever-growing violence she saw around her. She draws inspiration from women like Ingrid Newkirk, founder of People for the Ethical Treatment of Animals (PETA), and Julia Butterfly Hill, founder of the Circle of Life Foundation—women she feels are leading us into a new society "where kindness, compassion, and the sacredness of all of life (the Earth) is emphasized."

Sharon's integration of self-reflection and purposeful action is a yoga that offers inspiration to us all. She never misses an opportunity to get her message across and, although it may take some by surprise when she speaks her truth, the power and clarity of her words bring the point home: we are not separate. "All the great teachers in history were radicals. When those last few moments come, we don't want to regret

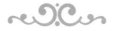

that we didn't take up those opportunities to speak and stand up. Theory is good, but it's useless unless you can apply it."

———————————

SHARON GANNON is cofounder of the Jivamukti Yoga Method, which integrates asana practice with an ethical lifestyle focused on attaining enlightenment through compassion for all beings. Sharon codirects the Jivamukti Yoga Center in New York with David Life, and she is the author of *Cats and Dogs Are People Too*; *Jivamukti Yoga*; and *The Art of Yoga*.

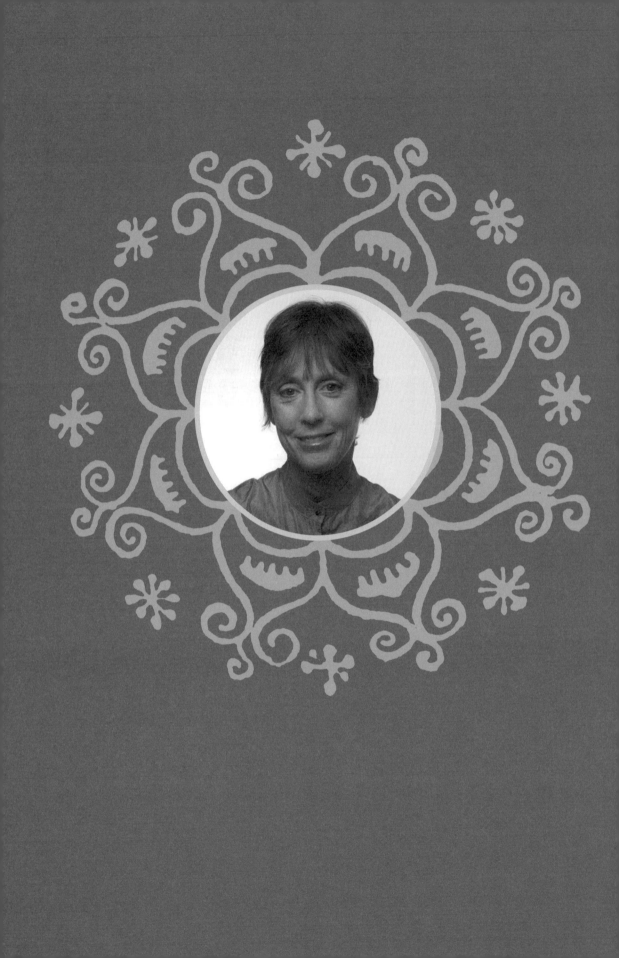

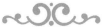

SALLY KEMPTON

Swami Durgananda

*Meditation allows you to carve out a
relationship with the inner presence that is the
deepest part of yourself. Eventually,
you find that you can rest in that presence
through the storms of life and so that
everything you do comes from the awareness
that that's who you are.*

At the age of twenty-six, while sitting in her living room in New York listening to the Grateful Dead, Sally Kempton had an ecstatic experience of love emanating from every part of the room and every pore of her being. This experience—a jolting contrast to how she had seen reality her whole life—gave her a taste of what was possible. She wanted that feeling again. Though she knew she might be perceived as "softheaded" by her left-wing political friends, who were suspicious of people who started by advocating for social change and ended up as spiritual seekers, she stepped onto the spiritual path. This path has led her to become one of the most sought-after meditation teachers in the country.

It was the early 1970s when Sally began her search for alternative ways of experiencing the world. At the time, she remembers that everyone on the spiritual path was "engaged in pretending to be Indian," with the men walking around in *lungis* and the women wearing *saris* (traditional Indian clothing). She closed the door on her life as a writer when she joined some friends involved in Arica, an integral body-mind-psyche-spirit meditation system developed by Bolivian teacher Oscar Ichazo. She moved to Los Angeles and started teaching for Ichazo's organization. While there, she started having dramatic energy experiences. During one period of intensive meditation, she recalls, her awareness shot up out the top of her head and light poured into and filled her body. "It was incredibly wonderful and really scary," she says. "In that moment of grasping for something to hold onto in the general dissolution and delight, I inwardly heard the name Swami Muktananda."

On Swami Muktananda's first visit to the United States in 1970, Baba Ram Dass (Richard Alpert) introduced him to the growing American spiritual community. Sally had heard about Swami Muktananda, the spiritual head of the Siddha Yoga lineage, from friends, who described him as a "real traditional-style guru who could transform your consciousness through his presence." He was also known as a master of *kundalini* energy; when Sally met him, she reexperienced the explosive energy she had felt in that initial awakening of love that had drawn her to the spiritual path. "An explosion occurred in my heart . . . his transmission was like that for many people, essentially a heart-to-heart blast of love-energy." Like many in the growing Siddha Yoga organization, Sally found in Swami Muktananda a catalyst for healing deep wounds. "The naturalness, and unconditional quality of the love he generated made living around him quite ecstatic. Often, it felt as if I were moving through a honeyed landscape of unconditional affection and regard." After Sally spent several months serving and studying with him, she felt she had to decide whether to return to her old life or start a new one.

She decided to go back to her career as a writer, and live as a "normal worldly person who also did spiritual practice." She spent an afternoon calling editors and got an assignment from the *New York Times Magazine*. She was feeling rather satisfied that her skills were still in demand. But then she realized that Muktananda was sixty-nine and wouldn't be around for long. "I saw that I had a unique opportunity to study with a powerful guru, and I wanted to continue the process I was in with him." She made an agreement with herself that she would eventually come back to the "world" and take up her personal life again.

She spent the next few years traveling around the United States and India with Muktananda. After eight years of touring with him and living at his ashram in India, she was ordained as a swami in 1982. She took vows to give up worldly ambition and spend her life in service to the divine. She then returned to the United States, and spent twenty-one years teaching Siddha Yoga at the organization's ashrams on the East and West Coasts.

Although Swami Muktananda was "like a big cosmic father," and had the capacity to make everyone feel deeply loved and seen, as a traditional Indian guru is known for doing, he also had a fiery personality and demanded intense discipline in his students. "In the traditional guru/disciple contract, there's an implicit agreement that as a disciple, you commit yourself to fully serving and following the guru's instructions, and the guru in return promises to kill your ego, take away a big pile of your obstructive karmas, and show you who you truly are," says Sally. "But it's not a magical quick fix, in any sense of the term." She acknowledges that in contemporary Western society, where so many people have parental issues, there is often a lot of projection, especially when the teacher is highly charismatic. Students can project onto the teacher their own needs and dependencies, their spiritual concepts and ideals. Sally feels that this process is part of the spiritual journey, and that one of the tasks of a guru is to refuse to accept those projections. In other words, the guru throws our projections back at us, and this forces us to own them. Unfortunately, not everyone understands that this is part of the process, so people often suffer intensely when their projections aren't realized. "You might have an expectation that the guru will be the perfect parent or friend or even deity, but a guru rarely behaves in the way we expect. When people don't understand this, they often end up feeling unhappy with the path or with the teacher."

A self–described "father's daughter" (her father was Murray Kempton, a Pulitzer Prize-winning news columnist), Sally admits she wouldn't have accepted a female teacher back then. In any case, at the time there weren't many female role models for a spiritual seeker. "For me, both intellectual and spiritual prowess were masculine qualities," she says. While Sally identified with her father and aligned herself with that energy in her life as a writer, she used her own intellectual prowess to rebel against male authority. In "Cutting Loose," an article published in *Esquire* in 1970, she reveals her conflicted relationship to the masculine, alternately confessing her dependency on men and raging against their supposed superiority. Around that time, she also took part in a sit-in against the *Ladies Home Journal* and appeared on *The Dick Cavett Show* to confront *Playboy*'s Hugh Hefner.

Ironically, when she gave up her life as a writer to follow her spiritual path, it was still under the fold of the Great Cosmic Father—but it was also a journey that eventually led her to integrate the feminine: at the core of Siddha Yoga is the awakening of the *kundalini* energy, or *shakti*, which is identified as a feminine force and lies dormant within each of us. In her book, *The Heart of Meditation*, Sally writes, "the sages who compiled the Hindu Tantras, yogic texts in which *kundalini* is invoked and celebrated, regarded it as the living deity, *kundalini*, or *shakti*, the goddess, whose special gift to us is spiritual awareness." According to the Eastern texts, the *kundalini* energy, which revealed to Sally the vastness of her own nature, can be awakened spontaneously, through certain hatha yoga practices, meditation, and devotional practices, or through the direct transmission of energy through a guru. The Siddha Yoga lineage follows the Tantric tradition, in which *kundalini* is awakened by a *shaktipat* guru—one who has the ability to pass on their own state of self-realization to others. Swami Muktananda was such a guru.

When Muktananda died in 1982, Sally didn't feel she could simply walk away. Having taken the vows to be a swami, she was committed to doing his work, which meant serving the organization and supporting the structure that he had created. Interestingly, Muktananda's closest disciple was a woman, Swami Gurumayi Chidvilasananda, and she took the seat as spiritual head of the Siddha Yoga lineage after his death. Unlike Muktananda, Gurumayi was not a traditional yogi. She grew up in Bombay, attended college, and was interested in the social and relational aspects of spiritual practice, as well as its inner dimensions.

Having lived with one teacher of each gender for over thirty years, Sally reflects on the differences. "What Muktananda taught me was to put aside the identification with the body and personality, to focus on the unchanging, the unborn. He put intense emphasis on the importance of finding God inside," which Sally considers a traditionally masculine approach to yoga: transcending or ascending out of the personal to experience enlightenment. "He taught that the world is also part of the divine, but the example of his life convinced me that to follow the path meant to reject worldly concerns and simply focus intensely on inner practice." Gurumayi, on the other hand, was extremely concerned with the way people lived their lives on a day-to-day level. "She was very much about, 'O.K., you have these realizations, but how do they apply to the way you treat other people? How do they apply to the way you do your work or the way you handle your health and your money? In other words, how do you make it all practical?'" Gurumayi also gave attention to psychological issues that weren't seriously addressed when Muktananda headed the organization, because she was more aware of how Western psychotherapy can play a role in spiritual practice.

Sally's own teaching naturally reflects the influence of both her teachers, as well as her own inner integration. "I always loved the teaching that the feminine is power, is *shakti*, is the creative impulse in consciousness. However, it took a lot of assimilation for me to own it." Sally sees the feminine as an energetic, feeling-based approach to meditation and yoga, rather than an approach that simply asks us to become the unmoved witness, or "the muscular warrior"; she considers the "energetic, dancing, shape-shifting" quality of the divine to be its feminine side. This dance is reflected in her life and teaching. "When I am most in touch with the feminine, I am very much operating through feeling—not emotion, but feeling as a quality of perception. In that mode, you work by taking in the energy of a person or group, and work with that energy, sometimes following and sometimes guiding its flow. But you're never out of touch with this feeling experience of the group or the environment; you're never trying to impose anything, or simply following an agenda. You're always feeling your way, finding how the energy can expand." In her own life, much of her work has been allowing herself to have emotions, rather than suppressing them, while at the same time not taking the content of them so seriously: to see through the drama of an emotional reaction into the energy behind it, and work with that.

Learning how to hold emotions without getting thrown off course by them is part of the work of meditation practice. "If we could say that there are gender-related pathologies, I'd say that the male is disconnection or dissociation. The female pathology tends to be emotionality. For most women I know, the path towards real empowerment and self-contentment often has to do with learning how not to identify with and merge with your emotions." Sally recommends going to the heart of the emotions, finding the energy there and letting it transmute itself. How? "Suppose you're feeling extreme anger or extreme fear. First recognize that the story, the tale that the fear or anger is telling you, is secondary." She encourages us to put aside the story and focus on the actual experience of fear or anger, how you feel it in your body, what the texture or energy of it is.

> Go deep into it. Feel the pure sensation of anger or the pure sensation of fear in your body. Stay with the feeling-sensation, which can be hard to do at first, because you will tend to go into the story or the description. If you can just stay with it, eventually the feeling of anger or the feeling of fear loses its sharp edges, as it were, and you begin to be aware of the energy behind it. The energy behind it is always a kind of love-energy or life-energy, and it always has a lot of strength and power because those extreme feelings

like anger or fear carry intensely condensed energy. This is the Tantric approach to emotion and it can lead to great states of realization—you go straight into the feeling until you come to the core of it and the core of it is *shakti*, love and energy.

Sally also recommends that her students use the many resources available to work with their psychological issues through psychotherapy and to access the muscle memory of stored emotion through bioenergetics and other modalities.

Today, living in California's Carmel Highlands, Sally has come full circle, integrating the transcendent practices of yoga and meditation with daily life. Having left the ashram in 2002 to live a life that was "less special and protected," she has returned to one in which she happily faces the same issues as everyone else and brings the meditation practices outside the ashram setting through her classes, workshops, and retreats. She has returned to writing, with a book, *The Heart of Meditation*, and a regular column in *Yoga Journal*. Her teaching now is about how to live your practice in "the nitty-gritty, day-to-day, often messy situations that life brings us." She says: "This is the work: fully integrating your practice into the way you think and the way you live. I find that it's always new, always challenging, and totally fun.

SALLY KEMPTON is one of today's most experienced and insightful teachers of meditation and spiritual growth. She offers heart-to-heart transmission in meditation through her Awakened Heart meditation workshops, classes, retreats, and yoga philosophy trainings. Her book, *The Heart of Meditation: Pathways to a Deeper Experience*, was published under her former monastic name of Swami Durgananda, and she currently writes a column for *Yoga Journal*.

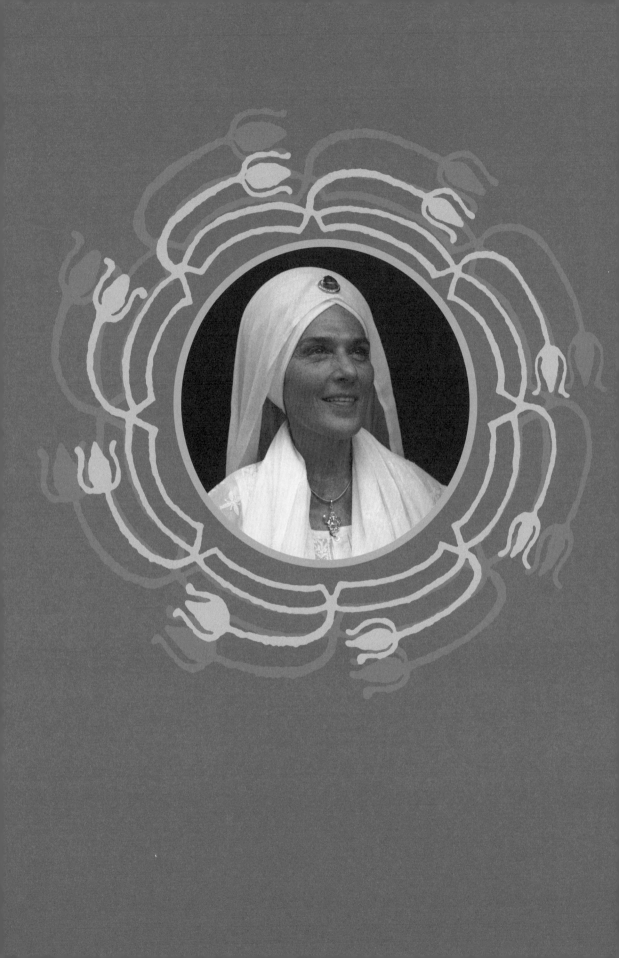

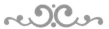

Gurmukh Kaur Khalsa

Yoga is self-acceptance
and self-love, not self-improvement.
You're perfect as you are.
To me yoginis must
declare self-love and be rebellious and
revolutionary—
because that's who we are.

*i*n her jeweled turban and willowy whites, *Kundalini* yoga teacher Gurmukh Kaur Khalsa floats into the room at the Omega Institute in Rhinebeck, New York. She comes across almost informally at first and when she starts speaking, there is not a hint of the intensity to follow. She draws us in slowly with meandering stories of her spiritual quest: living among the Indians in Oaxaca, Mexico, two carefree years as a hippie on a beach in Maui, meditating seven hours a day at a Zen center . . . the synchronistic flow of events that led her to *Kundalini* yoga thirty years ago. Soon, she leads the class in an unusual combination of yoga *asana* (postures), *mudras* (symbolic hand gestures), *pranayama* (breathing practices), and *mantras* (sacred words) designed to induce tranquility. Little do we know that by the time class ends we will have held an imaginary viewfinder in our hands and moved it back and forth, back and forth, until our arms felt like they were going to fall off; been transported to another realm through breathing and chanting; opened our arms like wings and "flown home" to ourselves. When we land we feel wrung out, cleansed, and renewed. "As we go along, you will lose the mind. Give the mind over to that bigger mind," she encourages. "Live in the infinite, rather than the finite," she says.

It's no accident that Gurmukh has a passion for sharing these teachings with women, particularly pregnant women. At twenty-one, she became pregnant by her boyfriend, and although they married, she went through a lonely and difficult pregnancy and a cold, clinical birth. It was 1964 and her husband wasn't allowed in the delivery room, where all eyes were on a television broadcasting the gubernatorial elections; she was given an epidural without her consent. Uninformed of her choices and lacking confidence, she followed the doctors' orders and became a reluctant participant in the Western medical model of childbirth. Her son, Shannon, was born with a congenital heart defect. He died seven months later. With no tools or ability to access her inner resources, she was at a loss as to how to deal with the pain, isolation, and guilt. Her marriage eventually dissolved and she set off on a spiritual search to understand why she was in the world and what her purpose was in this life.

After traveling for several years, Gurmukh thought she had found the answer to her search with Zen Buddhism. Just before she left for Japan to train as a nun, she ran into an old friend in Big Sur, California. He told her that God had come to him in a dream and assigned him the task of bringing her to an ashram in Arizona. Seeing it as part of her journey, she headed off with him in his Volkswagen bug. It was here that she met her teacher, Yogi Bhajan, the Sikh master who brought *Kundalini* yoga to the West. She had also found her spiritual home. Once there, Yogi Bhajan gave her the name by which she is now known, which means "one who helps thousands across the world ocean."

Although she knew she had found her path in *Kundalini* yoga, it wasn't until twenty years after Shannon's death, when Gurmukh gave birth to a healthy daughter, Wahe Guru Kaur, that her true mission in life became clear: to help women have a conscious experience of pregnancy and birth, make informed choices, and trust in their own innate intelligence. At the age of forty-three, she started by integrating Yogi Bhajan's practices into a prenatal yoga program for herself, which allowed her to deliver her child at home, with the help of a midwife. Word spread, and students started seeking Gurmukh's help with their own pregnancies and births. Today, at her yoga center in Los Angeles, Golden Bridge, Gurmukh and her coteacher, Devi Kaur Khalsa, an R.N. and childbirth educator, have a full family program where they teach everything "from the epidural to the family bed," as well as the emotional and spiritual work involved in preparing for birth and beyond.

Women often come to Gurmukh's popular pregnancy classes with the hope that practicing yoga will help ease the pain of birth. "Little do they know the rebirth they are going to go through," she smiles knowingly. While yoga postures help to prepare the body physically for birth, Gurmukh's classes take childbirth preparation to another level. According to Gurmukh, for every month of our own pregnancy, we relive the same month of being in our mother's womb. While some students' mothers sailed through their pregnancies and had positive birth experiences, others were depressed, drugged, had complications, or even died in childbirth. "They clear out their own birth through yoga so that they're free of that historical data and they don't have to repeat it."

Gurmukh encourages women to find out about their own birth and also to address any unresolved anger and resentment towards their parents that may arise during pregnancy. Specific meditations and mantras are given to heal emotional wounds and release past conditioning. "We have a lot of work to do, but they're so open to do it. And then they reincarnate a child who won't carry the same history." Meditation and chanting also help these mothers access their intuition and go beyond the mental concepts that can block them from their body's innate birthing intelligence. Gurmukh feels that women can help us heal the planet. "Because we are the ones who are bringing in the human race. We are the ones who can change in utero the karma and destiny of that soul." She uses the example of the Buddha to show how "one little man" can have such a powerful impact on the world.

Forty days after giving birth, the new mothers return for yoga with their babies. "We'll have fifty, sixty women, and maybe three sets of twins," Gurmukh says. She teaches these new mothers to "get their juices going," activating their glands and hormones through Kundalini yoga, helping them regain their strength through abdominal and Kegel exercises. Then they bring the babies into it. "We get up and dance—dance like crazy and we twirl and we sing." Equally as important as the yoga, Gurmukh emphasizes creating community. New mothers share cookies, tea, and conversation after class, and many form bonds that last a lifetime. "Community, community, community," she says. Gurmukh's favorite classes are women's classes, "because when women get together we're a hoot. We can drop our personalities and our concern about how we look. We don't have to be out there competing for jobs, competing for daddy's love. We can just hang out—we laugh, we play, we cry, we dance."

Each class ends with the mantra *Sat Nam*, which means "I am Truth." In *Kundalini* yoga, *mantras* are repeated over and over to bring about a shift in consciousness. Gurmukh emphasizes that when women say this *mantra* throughout their pregnancies, it anchors them in the breath, allowing them to experience the power of the breath beyond the power of the mind, which is incredibly helpful during childbirth. Gurmukh points out that most of us use *mantras* all day long, often unconsciously, both out loud and silently to ourselves. "'It's never gonna work, I'm tired, I should, I can't, I sure hope it's gonna work.' . . . It will just keep you caught in that law of cause and effect and cause and effect."

According to Gurmukh, not only is it important to become aware of the words themselves, but also the way they are spoken. As a practice, she recommends letting anything come out of your mouth at first and simply notice what you're saying all the time. Gurmukh herself never uses the word "should" any more. "'Should' has a judgment on it; there are so many words that do." She feels that we've been so deeply conditioned to give our power over to an external authority—the state, the church, the medical institutions—and that this is reflected in our language, which in turn keeps us caught in that paradigm. In her classes, she often has women partner up, go for a walk, and share their ideal vision of themselves and their lives—not at some time far off in the future, but as if they were already there. "When you say, 'I am,' you empower yourself with self-acceptance and love. When you say 'I want,' you are saying, 'I am not enough the way I am.'" Sometimes, the best choice of words is no words. She tells the story of two sisters sitting next to each other on a park bench. They remain silent for a long time. "As they get up to go, one turns to the other and says, 'That's the best conversation I've had in a long time.'"

Gurmukh never thought she'd end up in a big city like Los Angeles, but she feels that the teachings are needed there. After teaching privately to celebrities, Gurmukh realized she could reach more people if she taught group classes and opened a center. Golden Bridge Yoga has become a thriving yoga center that hosts diverse events and offers teacher training. Her studio, which emphasizes chanting and meditation, is a bit different from most others in America. "What we're learning in America is really a men's yoga. 'Just do it, push through'. . . . Women are getting the testosterone rolling

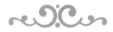

and they're being good gymnasts, but they're not getting fulfilled." She feels meditation is the essential ingredient that is missing in American yoga.

Gurmukh travels to India four times a year, so she is keenly aware that the emphasis on the physical aspects of the practice dulls in comparison to the spirituality that is celebrated in India. She feels that this focus on the physical can cultivate an environment where women compete and compare. She feels that this goes against our true nature, which is to embrace each other for who and what we are. "It's kind of crazy how the grace has gone out," she says. "At least they [many Western students] went to the gym and found yoga and now their soul is going to seek—now what, now what? And then they're going to go towards spirit. So there is a divine plan." As a result, Gurmukh sees that more and more women are leaning towards the teachings of the Mother, of the feminine aspects of the universe. "In the old days, the priest, the rabbi, and the state said 'this is the truth,' and then you mimicked it." Gurmukh feels we have to experience the truth for ourselves, and the only way she's found to experience the truth is through yoga and meditation. "And so we start small as yoginis, as teachers. We don't beat people up, we subtly teach it and give people an experience of it."

When Gurmukh first met Yogi Bhajan, he told her she would deliver babies. While living at his ashram in northern New Mexico she at first took this literally, thinking she would be a midwife. Now, thirty-five years later, she understands that he meant she would help deliver souls into the arms of conscious mothers, helping them prepare physically, mentally, emotionally, and spiritually to nurture these beings through life. "Yoga can deliver you home," she says.

GURMUKH KHALSA is the cofounder and director of Golden Bridge in Los Angeles. Since being baptized thirty-five years ago with the Sikh spiritual name meaning "one who helps people across the world ocean," Gurmukh has dedicated her life to fulfilling her namesake. For nearly three decades, students in Los Angeles and from around the world have sought out her classes in kundalini yoga, meditation, plus pre- and post-natal yoga. She has been married for twenty-two years to Gurushabd and has a twenty-one-year-old daughter, Wahe Guru Kaur, who also lives in Los Angeles. Gurmukh is the author of *The Eight Human Talents: The Yogic Way to Restore the Balance and Serenity Within You* and has produced the video *Kundalini Yoga with Gurmukh Kaur Khalsa*.

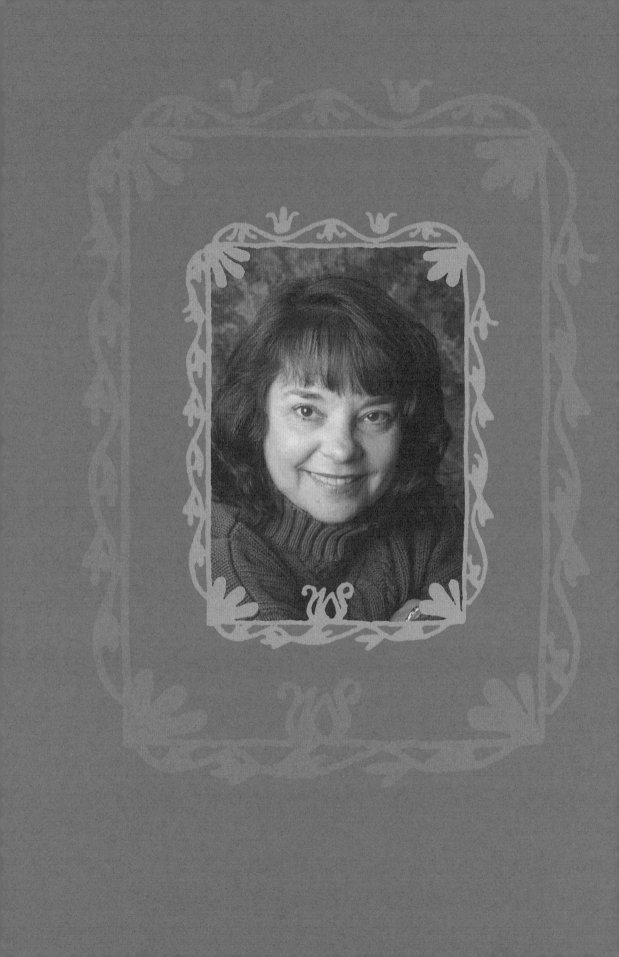

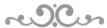

JUDITH HANSON LASATER

Above all, I want us to
remember that the way we step on the
mat is no different from
the way we live our life. There's absolutely
no difference. I bring my total
being to my practice. Do I push myself in
my practice? Then I push myself
in my life. I hope we can all evolve
into students who invite yoga
into ourselves, students who long to
become the yoga.

With five books and hundreds of magazine articles on yoga to her credit, Judith Hanson Lasater is rarely at a loss for words when it comes to the subject of yoga. A leading figure in the field of yoga in America for over thirty-five years, Judith is a founder of the Iyengar Yoga Institute in San Francisco, a cofounder of *Yoga Journal* magazine, and president of the California Yoga Teachers Association. With a degree in physical therapy and a PhD in East-West psychology, Judith seamlessly weaves anatomy, physiology, psychology, and philosophy into her teaching. Her in-depth approach to yoga extends into every aspect of life, including words we speak on a daily basis: "because I believe when you open your mouth, you change the world," she says. One of the foundational principles of yoga is *satya*, which means speaking the truth. When asked about her views on women in yoga, Judith clearly shares hers.

Judith expresses her concern about the ideal images of women seen in many yoga magazines today, with slim hips, slender thighs, and perfect breasts. She says these ideals negatively impact the modern yogini's perception of yoga practice. Most female bodies do not come close to these "ideals," and these images can feed into the feeling that we are not "enough" as we are. "Most women in our culture don't like their bodies, they don't like their breasts, they don't like their noses, their faces, and they're constantly telling themselves sentences that are self-loathing." In her classes and workshops, Judith sees how students take those beliefs to the yoga mat. "We inflict the poses on our body and we move at the speed and rhythm of the mind instead of the slower speed of the body." In the process, students miss the enjoyment of the practice and increase the potential for injury.

"Our culture doesn't honor just being present, but instead we honor doing, productivity, and action. And so where do we go now for rest and recuperation?" she asks. "We can't go to the mat now because it's like a gym, it's like a mini-gym." She sees nothing wrong in working out or in loving active practices, but feels they have taken over the space of rest and quiet, of introspection and ease. "My question for myself and for all of us is how do we find balance? Because despite all its other benefits, we are not going to find spiritual solace in working out. It feels good; you release lots of endorphins, but what about our spiritual hunger? Maybe we are confusing the exhaustion which comes from a hard workout with the dynamic balanced state of relaxation."

Restorative Yoga is Judith's answer to this dilemma—teaching people to rest very deeply as an integral part of their yoga practice. Consisting primarily of supported seated, reclining, and mild inversions and *pranayama* (breathing practices) that induce a state of deep relaxation, Restorative Yoga is the antithesis of the sweaty "power yoga" found in many yoga studios throughout the country. Restorative Yoga—bodies reclining over piled-high bolsters, blankets rolled under their necks, eye bags covering their eyes—may look like an adult version of nap time, but it goes much deeper. Judith has found an eager following through spreading the word of restorative work. Her book *Relax and Renew: Restful Yoga for Stressful Times*, which describes the principles and practice of Restorative Yoga, has become part of every serious yoga teacher's library, and her Relax and Renew teacher training workshops fill within hours of opening registration.

Judith sees rest as a way of expressing a feminine view of the body. "Practicing from the feminine means to connect to your receptive consciousness, and thus can be done by both men and women. And ultimately, if you look at the Yoga Sutras or at other yogic

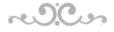

texts, they talk about the *sadhaka*, the seeker, creating a body/mind that is ready to receive the spirit of God. In other words, by practicing meditation, *asana*, *pranayama*, and self-study, we all—men and women—become the archetypal feminine to be able to receive God." She feels we've lost this understanding of practice today.

It's not just the overwhelming emphasis on the physicality of certain very active forms of yoga that Judith is concerned about. It's also the rigidity that can shape the practice, and the constant imposition of ideals from the outside. "What's feeling right to me, what's coming from me? This is an important question to continue to ask yourself during practice. If you put on yourself the ideal of pushing and power and challenge with no respite, your practice will become about achievement, just like the external world. I believe that many women cannot find themselves if they try to take that path; they will be more likely to lose themselves, in fact."

Judith's dramatic example of how women can benefit from Restorative Yoga is of a pregnant student who sought Judith's help because her baby wasn't growing. The woman was exercising excessively, trying to keep her abdomen as flat as possible during pregnancy. Her abdominal wall was thus not relaxing sufficiently for her uterus to grow and expand up and out of the pelvis, and as a consequence her baby couldn't grow. She was very muscular, with low body fat and wanted a "workout" that would help her. Judith gave her Restorative Yoga, saying, "I want you to go back to where you live and put on a sundress with no underwear. I want you to go out in the backyard and I want you to eat a juicy watermelon and let the juice run down your body so you get all sticky and sweet and I want you to sit in the sun and smell the sun on your skin. Stay there all afternoon with no watch and feel your juiciness. I really want you to juice up." The woman looked at Judith like she was crazy, "but that's what I felt she was lacking." Judith emphasizes that the real problem is never the practice, it's the attitude with which we practice, "which is not often about celebration, abundance, juiciness, health, and fullness. Sadly it's too much about controlling and austerity. When the Buddha sought enlightenment, the 'austerity stage' is the first one he tried and the first one he dropped."

"I have finally come to believe that men and women sometimes need very different things from the mat," Judith says. She points to the fact that in ancient times *asanas* were taught by men, for men. She also notes that yoga was taught to transform sexual energy to make it more available for self-realization. Partly because of the women's liberation movement, she feels that perhaps the pendulum has swung too far in the other direction and we no longer honor gender differences enough. "So what if you're pregnant, run a marathon! So what if you're pregnant, do a headstand for twenty minutes!" She sees that women's roles have changed dramatically over the years, whereas men's roles have not changed that much. "Now we raise our daughters to be brain surgeons and full-time moms. No one asks a boy if he wants to be a surgeon or a daddy. So women choose both and it is extremely stressful. Please hear that I am not saying that women shouldn't follow their dreams. I did, but it is long overdue that we acknowledge that you simply cannot do it all, have it all, be all things to all people."

Years ago, a light bulb turned on for Judith. As a long-time practitioner in the Iyengar system, she knew that Mr. Iyengar instructed women to do a quiet practice during the menstrual cycle to keep their *apana* (downward-moving energy) quiet. Judith noticed that she began to look forward to her monthly cycle because of these quiet poses. "There was this voice inside of me that would say 'Oh good, I get to do a softer practice today because it is my period.'" She began to reflect on what it was she was doing in her regular practice that was creating this resistance to it, this longing for softness and ease.

During this self-reflection, the seeds of her understanding of Restorative Yoga were born. Judith began to weave in days of receptive practice with the active practice she already did. This deepened her awareness of her attitude toward her practice. Was she coming in the spirit of honoring and appreciating her being? Or was it from a place of wanting to feel special and better than others?

To facilitate this receptive quality in an active practice, Judith teaches people to move from the belly. "This is where their core wisdom lives." Referring to research in the book *The Second Brain* about sites in the abdomen and chest that respond to specific neurotransmitters in the brain, Judith says, "When we say 'I feel it in my gut,' we physiologically actually do! That funny feeling in your belly is an expression of your deep knowing and the physiological proof of the process and power of intuition. I call this process of inner knowing 'the belly brain'" (pointing to her abdomen), "and I call this the 'head brain'" (pointing to her head). "I think the head brain is very fast, but the belly brain is never wrong."

In her own life, it took Judith a while to reconnect with trusting herself. A lot of that had to do with becoming a mother. The process of becoming pregnant, giving birth, and raising three children made her reflect on the residue of her thoughts and actions that she was leaving in the world through her children. If she said a word in anger, she would hear the same word repeated back to her two days later. "I realized that I don't want to create that, I don't want to leave those *samskaras*, those tendencies in others. I began to cellularly understand that my actions and words were deeply interwoven into the lives of others, the life of the entire world. That was really helpful for me. It gave me lots of motivation to pay attention to what I was choosing at each moment."

Judith recommends starting every day with a twenty-minute *Savasana* (Corpse Pose). Why twenty minutes? Because it takes fifteen minutes physiologically for the human body to relax deeply and to shift into rest-and-recuperation mode. For Judith, more important than the physical pose is the spiritual aspect of Savasana. "Savasana is an altered state and that's where all the healing is. In that deep state, after relaxation is complete, you can hear everything, but nothing disturbs you. Everything feels far away; if a door slams, you don't jump. You don't react to the world, you're really receiving the moment fully as it is."

According to the teachings of yoga, the body is permeated with energy. *Prana*, the masculine energy, is an upward-flowing energy that resides above the diaphragm. *Apana*, the feminine energy, flows downward and resides below the diaphragm. Restorative Yoga balances these two aspects of energy so that the practitioner is neither overstimulated nor depleted. To facilitate this balance, Judith recommends that a full twenty minutes be practiced daily in Savasana. She also recommends doing Restorative Yoga one day a week, and then, once a year, practicing Restorative Yoga for seven days in a row for at least an hour each day. "Getting into a rhythm of restorative practice is important," Judith says. "Many of us have lost touch with our internal rhythm, and we're out of harmony with it. We need to do 'nothing' for a few minutes every day."

Judith came to yoga in her early twenties, seeking relief from arthritis; while attending graduate school in Texas, she tried a yoga class that was offered at the YMCA/YWCA. When the instructor left ten months later, she was asked to take over the yoga program and hasn't stopped teaching since. Immediately drawn into the practice of yoga as a whole, she began reading everything she could find about the philosophy of yoga. She studied Sanskrit, the Rig Veda, and the Yoga Sutras. "Many of us don't understand that *asana* is just a small part of yoga, and that the practice of yoga is about understanding the nature of the mind and becoming free from it." Once she found the practice of yoga through the door of asana, she studied physical therapy to become a more skillful yoga teacher and eventually continued on to get her PhD in East-West psychology at the California Institute of Integral Studies in San Francisco.

Even with her depth of study and substantial experience as a teacher over the years, Judith continues to reflect on and examine what the practice of yoga is and how it applies to life. "What I want people to have most in their practices is to be very curious. Practicing

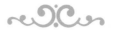

is all about being curious. What happens when I do this? What happens if I do that? What's arising in my mind? How is my breathing connected to my movement? Am I truly present and alive in this moment? What am I avoiding? What am I clinging to? Practicing thus becomes more about questioning than performing or having answers; it's more about being a little unsure. And that is what living life in the moment is all about, this willingness to be unsure and to step out anyway."

JUDITH HANSON LASATER is a yoga teacher and physical therapist who holds a PhD in East-West psychology. She has taught yoga around the world since 1971. She is married and the mother of three. Judith is the author of *Yoga Abs* (2005), *Yoga for Pregnancy: What Every Mom-to-Be Needs to Know* (2004), *30 Essential Yoga Poses: For Beginning Students and their Teachers* (2003), *Living Your Yoga: Finding the Spiritual in Everyday Life* (2000), and *Relax and Renew: Restful Yoga for Stressful Times* (1995), as well as numerous articles for *Yoga Journal* and many other magazines.

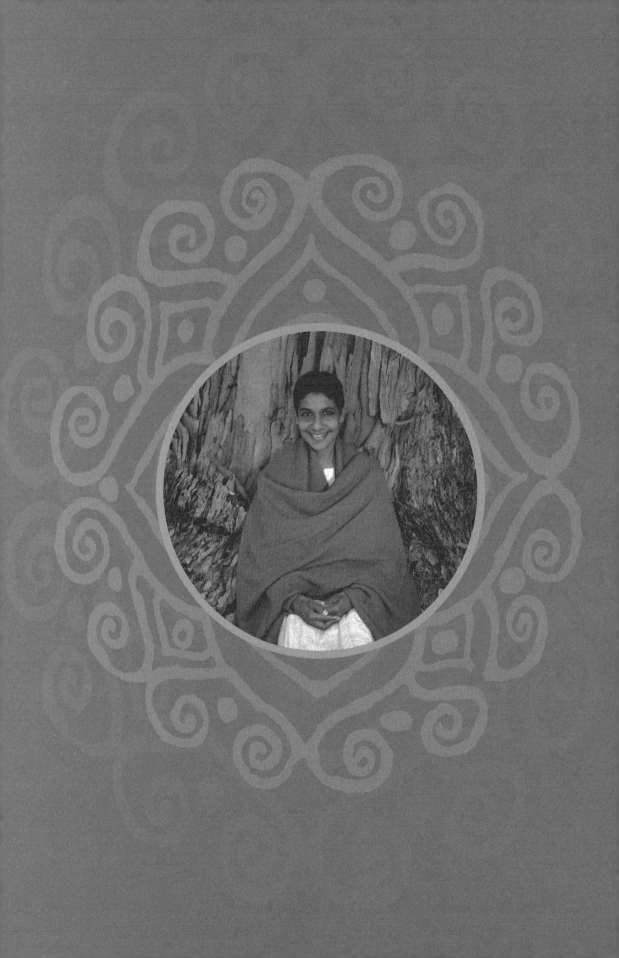

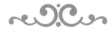

Sri Swamini Mayatitananda

Do less and wellness will be closer to you.

*I*f these yoginis sitting around the room at the Omega Institute have come for some relaxing yoga and a decadent spa treatment, they are in for a surprise. Sri Swamini Mayatitananda, a spiritual powerhouse in bright orange robes, is here to wake them up. "We have given over our Shakti rights," she booms. "We have handed them over to the institutions that 'care' for us." She nods to a devotee in white who acknowledges her signal and begins playing the drum. "Sit on the earth. Feel your joy as the Mother. Know that all healing happens here," she says, her arms sweeping out into the room. Sri Swamini Mayatitananda closes her eyes and sound pours from her mouth, "Aim, Hreem, Shreem, Kleem." (Kali, Lakshmi, Saraswati, Durga.) She is evoking the Goddess whose many faces gaze down from the walls of this conference center-turned-temple. The response is tentative at first. "Aim, Hreem, Shreem, Kleem." The sound of a didgeridoo vibrates into the space around and beneath us. "Aim, Hreem, Shreem, Kleem, Aim, Hreem, Shreem, Kleem." The energy builds as the call-and-response grows louder, stronger; bodies rise up and move. "Let your sound fly!" Sri Swamini Mayatitananda's ecstatic energy envelops the space.

Chanting in a room with Sri Swamini Mayatitananda is like plugging yourself into an electrical socket—everything lights up and comes alive. Through her substantial presence and her deep, resonant voice, she cuts through our "cosmic amnesia," as she likes to call it, reconnecting us to the life-giving force that exists within and around us. Affectionately called "Mother" by her students and disciples, Sri Swamini Mayatitananda travels extensively throughout the world sharing her unique "inner medicine" teachings, helping individuals, families, and communities take responsibility for their health and awaken to their own self-healing abilities. She reminds us that we are each a unique expression of the same divine maternal consciousness. Her call is to reclaim this creative feminine energy, to tap into our deep well of ancestral wisdom, and to expand our vision of who we are as women, sisters, mothers, and healers.

How do women today access our primordial feminine energy? "We must pause," says Sri Swamini Mayatitananda. "Society has given us strictures and scheduled structures that suffocate the life force." She says that our most important commitment must be to our own inner harmony and that only by taking time out from our daily activities can we access our intuition and recognize what is not harmonious. "That pause forces us to come to terms with all the junctures we have neglected along the way: the junctures of reconciliation, the junctures of contemplation, the junctures to digest and assimilate all that we have experienced." Pausing allows us to see where we are out of balance and helps us to recover our natural rhythms. "Life forces us to take pause when we do not take pause—through disease, divorce, separation, and dissociation," she cautions.

Sri Swamini Mayatitananda knows only too well the cost of being caught in the trance of modern life and losing connection to one's own deeper wisdom. At the age of fifteen, she left her East Indian immigrant family and a civil war in Guiana for New York to continue her studies, driven by the desire to carve out a new, independent identity for herself. Just eight years later, she had risen to the height of a successful career in fashion: boutiques bearing her name were in most of the high-fashion stores, and Hollywood celebrities wore her original designs. She kept up a frantic pace in an attempt to distance herself from her past. Like ninety percent of the women she now counsels, she ignored the underlying sense that something was wrong—until it was too late. By the time she finally went to the doctor, ovarian cancer had invaded her uterus and spread to other vital organs.

After enduring twelve major surgeries and countless radiation and chemotherapy treatments over two-and-a-half years, Sri Swamini Mayatitananda was told she had but two months to live. Realizing that she needed to reconcile with her past to facilitate her healing, she retreated to a cabin in Vermont where she fasted, dreamed, prayed, and had visions of her ancestors: priests who had been exported by the British in 1889 from their home in India to serve in Guiana as indentured laborers—uprooted, violated, and abused. She had spiritual visits from her estranged father, in which he read to her from the Hindu scriptures she studied as a child, the Baghavad Gita, and urged her to reclaim her life and fulfill her purpose. When she emerged from the cabin three months later, no sign of cancer in her blood or lymph nodes remained.

Through this process, she began to realize that her destiny was intricately interwoven with her illness. She recalls being in the recovery room after her hysterectomy, the doctor consoling her over the loss of her ability to bear children. "I already knew that it was more than not bleeding every month. It was really an understanding that my purpose in life was not to progress through the birthing womb, but the psychic womb." Another time she had powerful visions of Devi, one of the incarnations of the Divine Mother in the Hindu tradition, which she had honored during her childhood in Guiana. She later discovered through her own vision and experience that the Divine Mother provides each of us with the power to nurture and protect. Her healing presence sustained Sri Swamini Mayatitananda through some of the darkest times—and still inspires the work she does today.

"It's no mistake that cancer was one of my great gurus," she says. She reconciled with her family and, with the assistance of her father, eventually began studying the ancient texts on Ayurveda (Hindu science of health and medicine) and Vedanta (Hindu philosophy), particularly the portions of the Vedas dealing with healing and self-knowledge. After her father died, Sri Swamini Mayatitananda dreamt of him sitting cross-legged with his back to her in his white priest's robe, performing a fire ritual. The body appeared to be her father, but when he turned around the face was not his. Two weeks later, a friend gave her a tape of Vedic chanting and on the cover of the box was a photograph of the man whose face she saw in her dream, Sri Swami Dayananda Saraswati, one of the few living masters of the traditional teachings of Vedanta. Sri Swamini Mayatitananda recognized immediately that he was her teacher, and in 1986 she began studying with the great Vedic Master. She spent the following two years in his ashram, Arsha Vidya Gurukula, in Saylorsburg, Pennsylvania. She eventually accompanied him to India, becoming the first in her family in more than a century to return to the motherland.

Sri Swamini Mayatitananda has since visited India numerous times, spending ten years in *gurukulas*, ashrams that focus on the traditional student-teacher relationship, where her mentors were old monks and swamis with whom she sat, meditated, and "remembered" the work she now teaches. In the Vedic tradition, psychic transmission is honored as a tangible art of wisdom and incontrovertible means of study. In 1992, on the banks of the River Ganges, she was initiated in the Hindu tradition of her birth as a *brahmacharini*, a Vedic monk, vowing to preserve the ancient oral teachings of the Vedas and to helping others heal physically and emotionally. In service of this vow, Sri Swamini Mayatitananda relied on her cognitive memory, the collective knowledge that is available to us all when we "silence the mind and sit in the self" for understanding how these teachings related to her experience with cancer and how they could help others. Much of what she was studying in the Upanishads was reinforced and validated by her ancestral memory and her own intuition. In addition to the ancient Sanskrit texts on Ayurveda, the Samhitas of Charaka and Sushruta, Sri Swamini Mayatitananda has also studied the Atharvanas, original works of the ancient Ayurveda sages.

Through her studies and accessing her inner guidance, she unearthed long-forgotten practices that she now shares through her Wise Earth School of Ayurveda in North Carolina, her books on Ayurveda, and as founder of Mother Om Mission, a charitable organization that disseminates Wise Earth's unique inner-medicine healing education for at-risk communities. During the last twenty-five years, Sri Swamini Mayatitananda has worked unrelentingly with cancer patients and others who were considered terminally ill and trained more than five hundred practitioners and teachers who travel the world sharing Wise Earth's inner-medicine teachings.

Sri Swamini Mayatitananda believes the spirits of our ancestors provide us with guidance, inspiration, and protection, and play a significant role in our daily lives. She acknowledges and honors these ancestors through her spiritual service, which is the central theme of everything she does. According to Sri Swamini Mayatitananda, maintaining a vital connection with the spirits of our parents, grandparents, and great-grandparents provides us the opportunity to stand tall on their shoulders, whereas if we forget their presence, we "carry them on our backs," as she learned through her own experience with cancer.

In 2002, Sri Swamini Mayatitananda took her *diksha*, or Swamini initiation, during which her birth name and *karma* were cremated in accordance with Hindu rites. She has since been known as Sri Swamini Mayatitananda. Today, her energy is so vast and powerful that living beings around her seem to spontaneously heal. For example, when she moved to Wise Earth Monastery in the idyllic setting of the Pisgah Mountains, the cows in the neighboring fields had been suffering a devastating bout with a persistent eye disease. Just a few weeks after Sri Swamini Mayatitananda began chanting *Om* to them, the eye disease miraculously disappeared. She teaches that we all have access to this vast healing power within ourselves.

Sri Swamini Mayatitananda encourages women to take a proactive role in their own healing process. "As you change your inner rhythms, notice if the other parts of your life don't flow," she says. In her book *The Path of Practice, a Woman's Book of Ayurvedic*

Healing, she outlines *sadhanas*, practices that "replicate the sacred in nature through everyday activities that bring us into harmony with the great cycles of the cosmos and that reconnect us to that which is divine in us: our power to heal, serve, rejoice, and uplift the spirit." These practices stem from her early experience growing up in the 1950s in British Guiana, where her family kept their ancient rituals intact, living close to nature's rhythms. Centered on food, breath, and sound, the practices echo the rhythms of the kitchen of her childhood—grinding spices, pounding grains, sifting beans—movements that stimulate the natural rhythm of the heart and still the mind.

She also teaches women instructors to guide other women in how to harmonize their inner rhythms with those of "mother moon": menstruating with the new moon and ovulating with the full moon to heal physical, mental, and emotional imbalances. Under her guidance, thousands of women have learned *mudras* (sacred hand gestures) and *pranayama* (breathing practices) to realign their menstrual cycles with those of the moon. She remembers as a child when the women would gather and bathe in the light of the full moon, cultivating their connection to this lunar energy. According to Sri Swamini Mayatitananda, we carry the cellular memory of our mothers, our ancestors, and the wisdom of the divine mother in our wombs. Imperative to our health is healing and restoring our relationships with our mothers. We "carry their joys, pains, and cellular memory" which can manifest as blocked emotions or blocked life force, limiting our ability for expression in our lives.

Although much of her work has been transmitted to women, she says men will benefit as well. "If the woman gets it, the family gets it; the sons, the fathers, the husbands." According to Sri Swamini Mayatitananda, a man and a woman each have their own proactive energy distinct to their gender; each gender supports a specific archetypal energy. For men, it is the Shiva energy that is more alive in them. In the Vedic tradition, Shiva is the primordial male energy, the unmanifest consciousness, and is "the underlying supporting platform upon which Shakti resides." Shakti, the primordial feminine energy, is the dynamic force through which manifestation occurs. "The Shakti energy is more proactive in a woman than a man, because she can give birth." Sri Swamini Mayatitananda emphasizes that we all carry both of these interwoven powers within us and that the purpose of yoga is to unite these two principles.

"We need to stop defining ourselves as female/male, feminine/masculine, matriarchal/ patriarchal, maternal/paternal. It sets us up for the dualistic backlash." This confusion about roles was evident to Sri Swamini Mayatitananda at a meeting with her female colleagues to discuss the Women's Initiative of World Spiritual Leaders in Geneva, Switzerland, in 2003. Although many of the women wore business suits and carried laptops, still they were talking and thinking about how to be women, how to be feminine. She laughs her deep, joyful laugh at the memory of it. "We cannot do it through the mind," her voice drops, "it will not work. It's like working backwards . . . we have to remember. The clearest thing I can share with you is that gem. We don't access our incredible bounty of consciousness unless we know that the Mother consciousness is far vaster, far greater, far more all-generating and all-encompassing—infinite, as it were—than the feminine or masculine in ourselves."

SRI SWAMINI MAYATITANANDA (formerly Maya Tiwari) is a preeminent spiritual teacher who has transformed thousands of lives with her healing presence. Affectionately called Mother, she is a nurturer, healer, and educator—transforming disease and despair into health and inner harmony. Mother belongs to India's prestigious Vedic lineage, Veda Vyasa. She is the spiritual head of Wise Earth School of Ayurveda in the United States and the founder of Mother Om Mission (MOM), a charitable organization in Guiana, South America, whose pioneering inner-medicine healing education for at-risk communities is transforming violence and disease into harmony and health. Mother has written *The Path of Practice; Ayurveda Secrets of Healing* and *Ayurveda: A Life of Balance.*

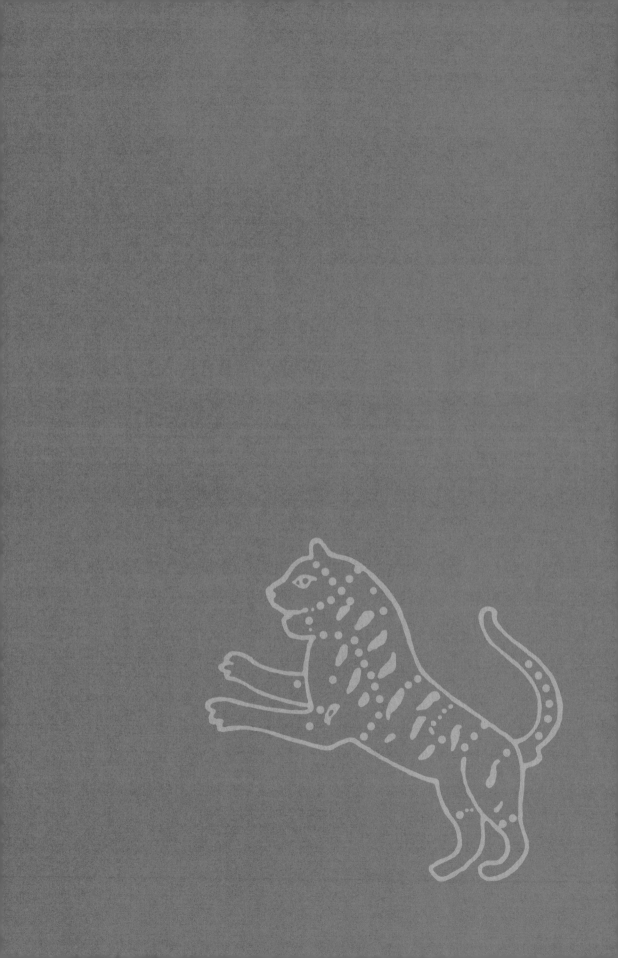

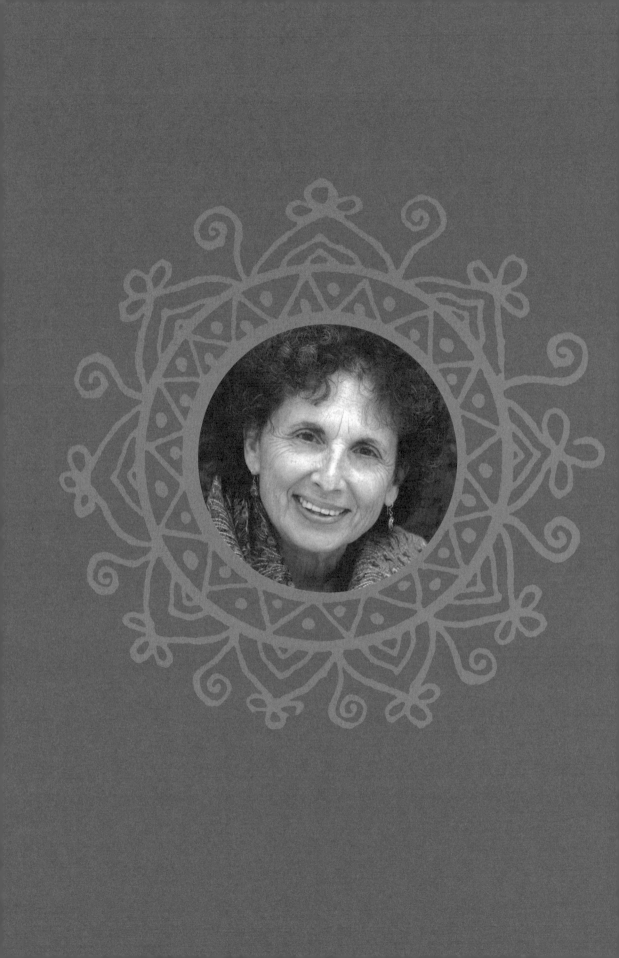

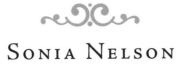

SONIA NELSON

*Chanting helps to sustain my link with nature
as something I am part of rather than
something separate from myself. Especially
now, with so many distractions in life, we need
to engage in some action that brings our
awareness to these deep connections.*

Chanting in a room with Sonia Nelson is like being transported to another realm, one where gods and goddesses are exalted and the earth, sun, and sky are honored. With Sonia, there is no mistaking the interconnection between the body, the breath, and the mind that gives voice to these sacred sounds. Simple universal gestures, like extending the arms toward a "higher force," or bringing the hands to the heart, as the place where our highest self resides, reinforce the connection to the chants, to nature, and to all of life.

How did this American woman from Philadelphia become one of the foremost teachers of a tradition that had been primarily the domain of Brahmin priests for thousands of years? Something transformed her in 1975 while she was sitting in a hotel room in Delhi listening to tapes of chanting. "I didn't really know what the chants were.

At that time I didn't even know what the Yoga Sutras were, but on hearing it, I felt an instant connection." The chanting turned out to be of Patanjali's Yoga Sutras. Although Sonia had traveled to India with her husband to study yoga, mainly as the practice of *asana* and *pranayama*, hearing those mysterious chants moved her life in a new direction. Thirty years later, finding a way to make these sacred sounds relevant to Western practitioners has become the primary focus of her work.

Today she teaches classes and workshops on chant and yoga around the country; she has also created instructional CDs for reciting hymns of the Vedas (the oldest Sanskrit texts from India) and the Yoga Sutras. She even attracts Indian-born students who come to study with her in Santa Fe at the Vedic Chant Center she directs. "They wonder themselves at how they, as South Indian Brahmans, are learning Vedic chant from an American Jewish teacher!"

For Sonia, bringing life to these ancient teachings and practices for our modern age is an ongoing exploration. "I am always looking for a common thread, universal themes that we can all relate to." She focuses on chants concerning the interrelationships among human beings, the environment, and the forces of nature, which bring our awareness to the sun, moon, earth, air, fire, and water. Her approach is both practical and powerful. When the chants involve the praise of gods and goddesses, she teaches them in a way that evokes the qualities that we as human beings need to aspire to, such as strength, energy, clarity, compassion, friendship, protection, support, and stability. In Vedic chant, reciting in praise of a particular force, whether it is a god, goddess, or a force of nature, links the chanter to these qualities. "I am fascinated with how bringing the mind to certain qualities through chanting keeps me more connected, more aware—not just of nature as something outside of me, but of myself as a part of it."

Listening to Sonia chant by heart multiple lengthy, complex verses that loop back and build on each other, the potential for sharpening one's mental acuity is clear. For Sonia, however, chanting is not only an intellectual exercise. Chanting engages the abdomen and lungs, awakening sensation in different parts of the body. "After attempting to breathe in completely while chanting, many women notice that they are unconsciously holding in their belly—a strong social conditioning—which keeps them from experiencing a full and relaxed breath." One of the most frequent comments she hears from female students, especially those who have given birth, is that chanting makes them realize how disconnected they were from their lower abdomen and how much they appreciate reestablishing that connection.

Sonia says that many women are drawn to chanting in a group for the feeling of community this creates. "It's a special kind of communication that comes alive by sharing our voices with others in the context of words that have a sacred quality." Sonia notes that yoga practice is a fairly solitary activity, even when we're doing asanas in a group setting. In her teaching, she emphasizes the relational aspect of chant and has moved away from using printed texts and handouts. While she acknowledges that words in print are helpful, especially when chanting a long passage, she finds that chanting from memory or by listening to one another and repeating what you hear creates a different relationship between people. "Students listen to me, taking something in. Then I chant, giving something back." She may also split the group up and have them chant and repeat to each other. "So the relationship is not just between the student and teacher, but from one student to another with a feeling of giving and receiving."

At a recent workshop on the Yoga Sutras, Sonia had each woman give a presentation on a sutra, relating it to her own life experience. One woman spoke of the challenges of raising a child with special needs. Another woman lost everything in Hurricane Katrina. They explained how the practical wisdom of the Yoga Sutras acted as a stabilizing force in challenging times. "It was a powerful and healing experience for all," Sonia observes.

Chanting gives some women new confidence to project their voices in a way that had been difficult in everyday communication or in public speaking. "You have to open your mouth in order to chant, so you become aware of any tendency to clench your jaw." This awareness extends to breathing and the unconscious habits that inhibit the breath, which is reflected in the way the sound comes out. "It is interesting that one of the sounds we use most frequently to encourage the feeling of the mouth being open is 'ma,' the universal syllable for mother."

Sonia's familiarity with the sound of foreign languages started in childhood, as both her mother and grandmother spoke Yiddish. When she was growing up, she spent years in a Jewish cultural education program, where boys and girls chanted in Hebrew to prepare for their bar or bat mitzvahs. Perhaps these early experiences, as well as her early interest in folk music, made her particularly receptive to Vedic chant.

The sounds drew Sonia in, but it was her teacher, TKV Desikachar, who took her deeper into understanding their healing wisdom. While her own study of Vedic chant was very traditional, through a one-to-one student-teacher relationship, Desikachar always modeled and encouraged her to adopt an innovative approach to teaching. A key theme in the art of adaptation is to refrain from imposing your ideas on another, and Sonia feels that cultural relevance is extremely important. When teaching meditation to students from diverse religious backgrounds who may not be receptive to practices from other cultures, Sonia uses an object of meditation from their own spiritual tradition, such as an image of Mary or Jesus in the case of Christians, or simply a favorite photograph of the natural world. Rather than reciting in Sanskrit, she may have the student learn chants in Latin, English, or Hebrew, with content ranging from biblical passages to poetry. The structure and general components of these practices are linked to those of the Vedic tradition. Sonia may suggest to students that while they recite a mantra, they place their hand(s) on different parts of the body, to direct the effect of the mantra to that place.

"If I'm chanting in English, I know what it means and it has one effect." Yet, when chanting in the original language of the chant, there is another effect that cannot be duplicated. "Sometimes when I'm chanting, I know what the words are saying; sometimes I have only a vague idea; and sometimes, no idea at all." For some students, the act of chanting itself produces a profound effect, and the meaning is secondary. For others, it is important to have at least some way to conceptualize the meaning of the chant.

Different chants have different qualities, and Sonia finds women especially sensitive to this fact. Some chants are fiery and have high energy, while others are softer and more melodic. With the many demands women have on their energy today, Sonia realizes that at different times we may require "more energetic chanting to wake us up and bring mental focus, while at other times we may need chants that are calming and soothing."

It was actually Desikachar's father, Sri Krishnamacharya, who began encouraging women to participate in Vedic chanting in India, during a time when this was not considered appropriate or acceptable. "He felt that women had a major responsibility to fulfill regarding the preservation and continuation of the highest values in society and this included carrying forward Vedic chant to future generations. He reversed his own traditional upbringing and began teaching women Vedic chant." Indeed, today the Veda Vani Chant Center in Chennai (Madras), India, has a female director and a faculty that is ninety percent female.

In 2003, when Sonia brought a group of students to India to study with Desikachar, he arranged for four groups of priests to chant for the students. At the end of each program, Desikachar asked Sonia's group to chant. "The priests were very appreciative of our interest in their tradition and some expressed their amazement that we could chant so well from memory. There wasn't a hint of resistance to these American women chanting the Veda." The fact that these priests were so open to hearing women practice this ancient tradition inspires Sonia.

Although Sonia did not have a female teacher, her close friend Mary Louise Skelton, who was also a mother, wife, and teacher, was an important role model for her. Mary Lou studied with both Krishnamacharya and Desikachar and was influential in bringing their teachings to the West through publications and programs associated with Colgate University. "Mary Lou was an extraordinary woman who was able to live a life of compassion that supported family, friends, and students, while maintaining high standards in all of her relationships."

Sonia's individualized approach to teaching is central to her work. Many students come to Sonia seeking help for a variety of physical and psychological problems, including breathing difficulties, anxiety, and depression. "Fundamentally, what the student is hoping for is to come out of *dukkha*, or suffering." Sonia takes into account the student's health, stage of life, type of work, family and social obligations, and interests. "The teacher's role is to see each student clearly, to see her situation and her potential objectively." The student also has a role: to be willing to listen and learn. "Our Western upbringing encourages independence and self-reliance and that sometimes gets in the way of receptivity." At the same time, Sonia recognizes that as a teacher, it is important to give only what is asked for. She refers to the exchange between Krishna and Arjuna in the Bhagavad Gita: "Krishna was Arjuna's chariot driver until Arjuna asked for help; at that point Krishna assumed the role of the teacher and began to teach Arjuna."

Sonia has thought a lot about the student-teacher relationship, and believes that being a student is more than having someone to help with asana practice. "Being a student means I am in a relationship with someone who can see, give direction to, and guide my potential." This relationship develops over time, and "becomes refined through the clarity of the teacher, the receptivity of the student, and the patience of both. There is a beautiful word in Sanskrit, *shradda*, faith, trust. These are developed over time and grow through the relationship itself." Sonia believes that if a teacher has faith and confidence in the source of her own teaching, this will be transmitted to the

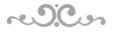

student, since, "the goal of the teacher is to help students discover their own nature, to help them move beyond their lack of clarity." Ultimately, however, the teacher is within. "The external teacher is always moving in the direction of helping the student to become their own teacher."

Sonia Nelson, director of the Vedic Chant Center, has been a student and teacher of yoga and Vedic chant for over thirty years. Her formal studies began in 1975 with TKV Desikachar in Chennai, India. Sonia has developed an approach for teaching Vedic chant to Western students and trains teachers to bring Vedic chant to a wider population. Sonia gives seminars and workshops around the country and at her Vedic Chant Center in Santa Fe, New Mexico. She has released a number of CDs and is recording a series of Vedic chant tutorials.

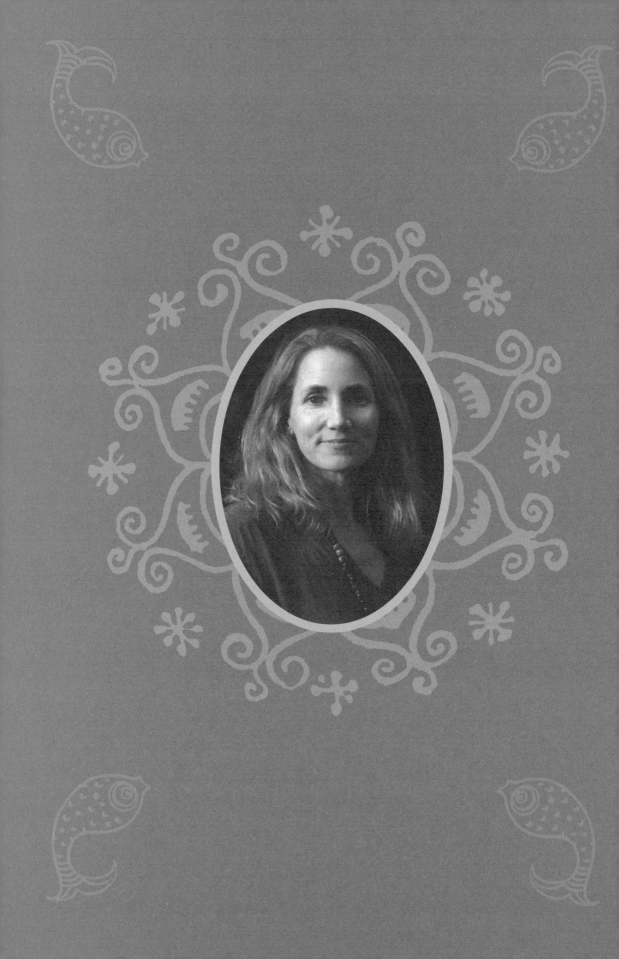

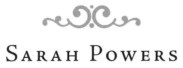

SARAH POWERS

I think we need the wisdom
teachings to continue to be interpreted and
shared by both men and women from a
multiplicity of ethnicities and backgrounds.
Our political as well as spiritual
leaders have been predominately
male for centuries, and both domains are out
of balance. It is vitally important
that we empower and embrace skillful women
leaders to help us integrate the
much-needed feminine principles of shared
community, radical tolerance,
and discriminating wisdom into our hearts,
as well as into our society as a whole.

When yoga teacher Sarah Powers arrived for a three-week retreat at a Burmese Buddhist monastery to study meditation with a male-female teaching team, she was disappointed to find that the female teacher had not shown up. Disappointment turned to discomfort on the second day when she took her place in the formal procession going into the dining hall—at the end of the line. Monks went first, and then Western laymen, followed by nuns. Western laywomen came last. "I felt that this was blatant sexism," she says. "I felt by lining up, through my complicity, I was agreeing with the situation."

Although she understood that the teachings, like yoga itself, are gender-free, she also knew that these traditions came through systems that were compiled, written, and taught by men. Sarah was aware that as a nonmonastic Western woman, her participation was in itself an advancement. So rather than trying to convert these institutions or conform herself, Sarah drew on the underlying principles of Buddhism and now weaves them into her practice and teaching. "In the Tibetan tradition, the feminine principle is described as the 'wisdom aspect' of our nature. I felt like this is a necessary and important element to add to the ever-present, active masculine principle." Her teaching integrates both aspects of practice. She travels around the world giving workshops and retreats on Insight Yoga— her synthesis of dynamic, flowing yang postures; long-held, passive yin postures; and silent meditation, supported by talks on the Buddha's teachings.

Sarah took up yoga in 1986 as part of her graduate studies at the Institute of Transpersonal Psychology in California. With a keen interest in integrating Eastern and Western practices, she honed in on the potential for self-transformation in the yoga class. During this period, in the late 1980s, group yoga classes were just beginning to take root in Los Angeles. After a year of studying both psychology and yoga, Sarah chose to become a yoga teacher. She found that whether or not people went to therapy, the yoga class environment offered exposure to self-reflective practices that encouraged them to look inward.

Sarah's spiritual yearnings were supported early on by both her husband Ty, whom she met at eighteen, and her mother, a practicing Buddhist. She remembers calling her mother when she was younger, in a state of confusion. "She would say 'Sweetie, just sit down, be quiet, look within and listen to that voice.' I had such a restless and active mind. I would say to her, ever impatient, 'Mom, I sit down and I get quiet and there are so many voices. Which one should I listen to?'"

Years later, her entrance into formal meditation practice was motivated by her own suffering. With a generous offer of support from a philanthropic yoga student in Santa Barbara, Sarah and her family were poised to take an extended trip to India in 1992. They put everything in storage, quit their jobs, and embarked on the first leg of their journey, to New York, where they waited for the money to be wired. None came. With a broken promise and no financial base, Sarah, Ty, and their four-year-old daughter, Imani, were left to reconstruct their lives. They filed for bankruptcy and slept on friends' floors. The whole process lasted about a year. "It catapulted me into questioning the way wanting and grasping something can really pull us to a place of disconnection. And yet, we can still feel like it's motivated by positive sources."

Having read about Buddhism while in graduate school, Sarah understood that the primary tenets addressed greed, hatred, and delusion. "The fundamental afflictions described in the Buddhist dharma (teachings) were being acted out in my personal life. I started out with greed, hated how it ended up evolving, and came out of it fully confused." Although Sarah knew she was resilient and that she would eventually re-create her life, she realized her more self-reflective side needed to mature.

Feeling that yoga alone was not going to work on these deep-seated issues, she sought out further training when her family relocated to the San Francisco Bay Area. She wanted to learn how to observe the movements of her mind and understand how it hooked into belief systems and assumptions. "In the Buddhist community, I heard the psychologically based language that so clearly described the particular ways we unwittingly govern our lives, and how to wake up from that. I felt like I had come home."

At the same time that Sarah dove deeper into meditative practices, she ran into Paul Grilley, one of her yoga teachers from ten years earlier. She had studied with Grilley at Yoga Works, where she had also taught Ashtanga yoga. Through him, she reconnected with the practice of yin yoga: long, passively held postures that loosen the dense connective tissues of the body and nourish the meridians (energy channels). Rather than emphasizing alignment to deepen the pose, the yin practice allowed students to stay within their own inner experience. She felt it was a beautiful complement to the active style she already practiced. "It has allowed me to feel into my body without trying to change it. You learn to surrender and develop a willingness to feel, rather than promote a willfulness to change what is felt. You only go deeper if the body naturally releases and your emotional tone is willing," Sarah says.

For Sarah, there's been a natural, side-by-side progression of both the meditation and the yin yoga. "I've really found that the psychological disturbances at the root of our suffering can be accessed through a number of doorways." She recognized that the arising of patterns and the potential of seeing directly into their nature was very strong in Buddhist meditation—and yet also available in a five-minute yin pose. "We really drop into that place of yielding, of surrendering, of letting what is within us percolate through and be inquired into." She sees these practices as interconnected and complementary. For meditation practitioners, the physical and energetic practices can help prepare for sitting. For those more involved in yoga's physical practices, the Buddhist teachings and meditation can open them to deeper levels of awareness and insight. "I think as any practice matures, it becomes richer. The tendency to stagnate and cling to the techniques themselves is a potential pitfall for any of us."

Sarah began attending silent retreats with Buddhist teachers Jack Kornfield and Michelle McDonald of the Vipassana tradition; Toni Packer, who was originally in the Zen tradition; and from the Tibetan tradition, Tsoknyi Rinpoche, who has since become her primary teacher. Although Tsoknyi Rinpoche is male, she also seeks out female teachers whenever possible. "I really appreciate a teacher who transcends their gender, who's not overtly feminine or masculine, but who's integrated both sides of their nature. And if they happen to be having a feminine experience in this life, I feel that that is really going to help me relate to what their challenges have been." In some of the historical writings, Sarah discovered that the Buddha's wife, Yashodhara, was thought to have practiced yoga, then called temple exercises.

While in the past some Buddhists felt that renouncing worldly life to seek enlightenment was essential, Sarah is interested in integrating spiritual practice with everyday living. She has been inspired by contemporary enlightened women such as Dipa Ma (1911–1989). This ordinary housewife overcame profound suffering, including the death of her husband and two sons, which left her a single mother to a third child. Dipa Ma eventually became an extraordinary meditation teacher. She showed other Indian mothers how to support each other by sharing household responsibilities and childcare so that they could reap the benefits of retreat. Sarah Powers feels that with so many female teachers and practitioners in the West, women have the opportunity to create a similar community of support for each other.

"This culture trains each of us in this independent spirit, thinking that somehow vulnerability is equated with weakness instead of strength. It's important to recognize that we need each other and that we need guidance. I feel it is important to seek out women we trust and allow them to reflect our distortions back to us as well as model new possibilities. We will benefit from allowing people to play the role of mentor, of older sister, of spiritual friend." While much of yoga and meditation practice is considered an internal solitary pursuit, the idea of *sangha*, or community, is an essential element of Buddhist practice. Along with the Buddha (teacher) and the dharma (teachings), sangha is the third of the three refuges that support the relief of suffering. Indeed, cultivating relationships with

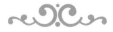

like-minded people has been integral to Sarah's life. She is aware of the isolation that can happen when we begin a spiritual practice, and says that these changes can create the feeling that nobody understands what you are going through.

Sarah also sees community as a mirror that reflects back to us when we get off track. In an article in *Yoga Journal*, she says: "Insight becomes wisdom only when it is rooted in the stream of your being, and that comes across in the way you relate. Without interaction, you really don't know who you are. It's especially important to have this reflection when you get confused and delusional." Sarah thinks the yoga community could certainly benefit from this idea. In the same article, she continues, "We could become a stronger group of people if we build a sangha that helps those who stray get back on the path, rather than damning them behind their backs. The Buddhist community does this, and it works." Sarah points out that connecting on a regular basis helps us all feel part of a greater whole, which reduces the tendency towards competition and what she calls "yoga fundamentalism"—the trap of getting caught up in feeling that one's own system or style of practice is somehow more elevated than others.

Recognizing the need for more connection within the yoga community, in 1989 Sarah initiated a yoga teachers' circle, inviting female yoga teachers to meet regularly to share their personal challenges, insights, and inspirations. This group of seven to ten women continues to meet today. Unlike a typical gathering with a lot of cross-conversation, the group begins by sitting in a circle for a thirty-minute silent meditation that creates a sacred space. Afterward, each woman has the opportunity to speak from her heart and be heard without interruption. The meetings end with shared food and conversation.

For her own personal practice, Sarah balances her energy between teaching, community activities, home-schooling her daughter, and working with her husband, who provides behind-the-scenes support for Sarah's workshops and retreats, as well as being a teacher himself. Sarah feels that setting aside time for daily practice is essential, as well as taking time periodically for deeper study and retreats. She has a three- to four-hour daily practice that includes Tibetan visualizations, active poses, yin postures, pranayama, and meditation. She goes on retreats three or four times a year for one to two weeks at a time. "You can't live a mindful life unless you also train in living mindfully, moment by moment. You have to have set aside time."

Sarah feels that the teachings need to be brought home, digested, and integrated into daily life to really have resonance for women today. Recently, she had the experience of being with a female dharma heir from a male lineage, the daughter of a famous meditation teacher. "She had so much power when she was being herself and interacting with the audience. I so appreciated that style of intercommunication and connectedness." When the woman began teaching within the model from which she was schooled, however, her energy shifted and her style became very dry and traditional. "She hadn't yet allowed herself to break free of the form; having been fed by that form, she had not yet let it translate into her own interpretations and rhythms." She was still conforming to a masculine model. This experience helped Sarah Powers reflect on her own journey with her male teachers. "I plan to continue to trust and value the way the teachings are going to come out through me, free of the authoritarian, pedantic cadence that can make points of view sound so unquestionable. That masculine style, shared by both genders, may cause some people to complacently accept what is being said, rather than allowing the teachings to support an investigation into their own experience, which is what breeds insight. The Buddha is famous for suggesting we not believe something just because we like the person saying it, or because it sounds true. Although we need ample exposure to wise guides, we each must take up the burden and the privilege of self-inquiry to discover true freedom."

SARAH POWERS began teaching yoga in 1987. She interweaves the insights and practices of yoga and Buddhism into an integral practice to enliven the body, heart, and mind. Her yoga style blends a yin sequence of long-held poses to enhance the meridian and organ systems with a flow or yang practice, influenced by viniyoga, ashtanga, and alignment-based teachings. Her main influence for the last seven years has been the Dzogchen teacher Tsoknyi Rinpoche. She teaches retreats with her husband, Ty, and together they home-school their teenage daughter, Imani Jade. They live in Marin County, California. Sarah is featured in the DVDs *Yin and Vinyasa* and *Insight Yoga*.

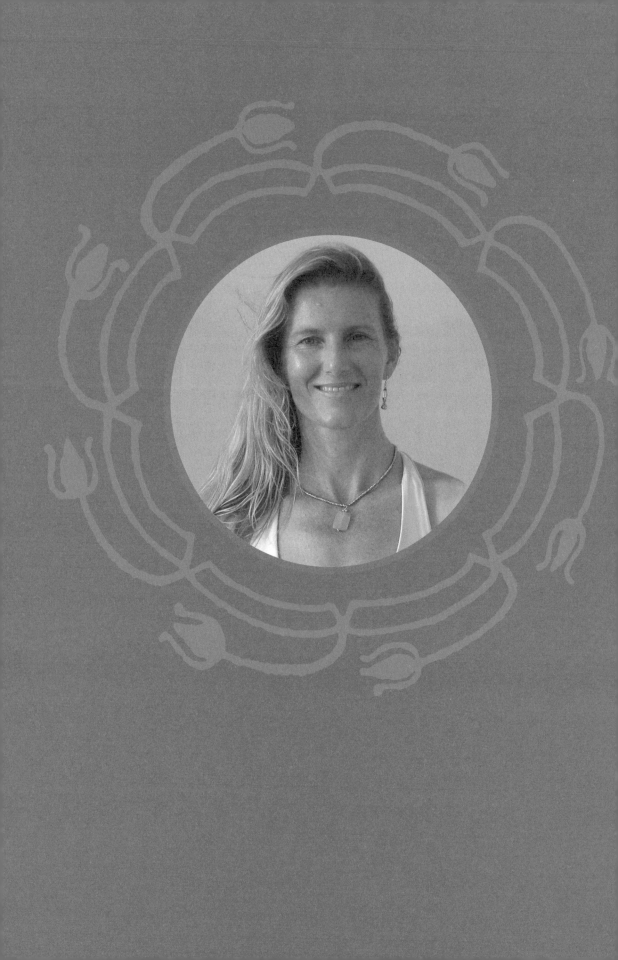

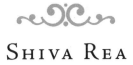

SHIVA REA

*The yogini is a woman whose
body has become her temple, her source
of discovery and renewal, the
place of remembering her life force.*

Blond hair flying in the wind, arms reaching skyward, her lean body arced in a backbend, Shiva Rea's dynamic images on her yoga CDs and DVDs reflect her state of perpetual motion. From New York to Los Angeles, Hong Kong to Costa Rica, Greece to South India, Shiva circles the globe teaching her juicy Vinyasa Flow Yoga and Trance Dance, inviting the world to get out of their heads and into their bodies to allow the creative life force to move through, inspire, and enliven them. Part yogi, part dancer, part river guide, this modern yogini echoes the sentiments of yoginis past who chose to forego austere asceticism for the body-positive, life-affirming practices of Tantra. A class with Shiva is a fluid journey through yoga, Ayurveda, and quantum physics that even the most steadfast tradition-alists may find hard to resist—the potential for full-blown ecstasy becomes available to those willing to loosen their grip on form and technique. "Don't push the river," she says, guiding us to ride the wave of the breath, the wave of the spine, the wave of our ever-changing experience; "it flows by itself."

For Shiva, the life force is not some abstract, New Age concept. While studying dance anthropology at UCLA's World Arts and Culture program from 1995 to 1997, Shiva wrote her master's thesis on hatha yoga as a practice of embodiment. However, when she became pregnant with her son Jai in 1998, Shiva's personal understanding of embodiment took on a whole new dimension. For ten years, Shiva had been a dedicated practitioner of the athletic style of ashtanga vinyasa yoga, a progressively more challenging series of flowing postures, and she assumed she would continue with the practice throughout her pregnancy. However, Shiva found herself slowing down and turning toward a more nourishing practice. "I kept telling myself 'Become the soil, become that deep, deep receptivity.'" For the first month of pregnancy, her asana practice consisted of lying over a bolster in the restorative posture known as Supta Baddha Konasana, or Reclining Bound-Angle pose.

Shiva recalls one of her teachers, Shandor Remete, telling her that when she was pregnant, she would learn more about the life force than at any other time. "It was absolutely true," she says. Slowing down, Shiva became aware of what an incredible *dharana* (concentration point) her growing belly had become. Having that lower anchor for awareness in the body, Shiva felt incredibly grounded. She laughs now at the absurdity of the idea she had of practicing ashtanga style with a big belly, with other pregnant women doing this strong, dynamic practice alongside her.

After Jai's birth, she resumed her ashtanga practice but found it was no longer a good fit. She noticed a "hierarchy consciousness" around the practice: "People acted like you weren't practicing yoga unless you were practicing ashtanga yoga," and it felt regressive to her. Although it took her several years to recognize that she was mentally conditioned to doing a set series of postures, an influx of visiting teachers from the Krishnamacharya lineage expanded her view. Through her studies in Ayurveda, she now understands that the heating ashtanga practice completely aggravated her *pitta-vatta* constitution (an Ayurvedic constitutional type which becomes imbalanced with too much heat, intensity, or fast movement). "It was just the wrong practice for me at a certain time in my life." After years of doing the sun salutations, which are foundational to the ashtanga practice, she started practicing moon salutations as well. She found that the cooling, calming movements that honor the rhythms and cycles of female moon energy balanced the heating, energizing aspects of the male sun energy. Adding these to her practice reflects how she sees her practice, or *sadhana*, as an integrative force, always relating to the "pulsation and polarity of solar and lunar as something that is natural and inherent." These changes in her practice and the "rejuvenation, nourishment, and initiation" of carrying her son directed Shiva to a more intuitive, feminine way of practicing and teaching.

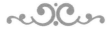

Shiva's father, an artist, loved the image of Nataraj, the dancing form of the Lord Shiva, and named his daughter after that deity. Her name was what initially drew Shiva to practice yoga. Like the god Shiva, who is seen as the first teacher of both yoga and dance, she is a true integrator. With her background in dance and various yoga traditions, Shiva's practice and teaching started to evolve after the birth of her son. Because of her experience at the age of sixteen working with a Tantric-based nonprofit organization in Africa (Ananda Marga), she found herself migrating toward Tantric practices, which recognize the creative energy of the universe as female, called Shakti. "Many of us were raised on a steady diet of the Yoga Sutras," Shiva says. Shiva broadened her studies to include Tantric texts as well, particularly the Vijnanabhairava Tantra, which teaches that the work of yoga is to spontaneously recognize our divine essence through the inner vibrations of the body. Shiva draws on the vinyasa teachings of the Krishnamacharya lineage, in which "postures are threaded on the breath like pearls on a string," Tantra; and dance. She sees dance as the spontaneous flow of Shakti that was at the heart of how yoga asanas came into being. "Every single source of energy on the yogic path in its essence is shown as dancing: Nataraj, Kali, Krishna, Ganesh." Some people in the yoga community have suggested that there might be a conflict between practicing yoga and dancing—as if they should not dance if they practice yoga. "I feel like dance is so important, and we know it's important because children dance, and they don't stop. And saints dance. Ramakrishna and Swami Satchidananda danced.

"What integrating elements of dance and Tantra did was totally fertilize my teaching of vinyasa. It's like being a classical musician and then leaving the orchestra and hanging out in New Orleans. All of a sudden jazz starts happening." Shiva deepened her understanding of Tantra with Swami Saraswati Sivananda of the Bihar School of Yoga and Tantric master Daniel Odier, a student of the Kashmirian yogini Lalita Devi. Although Shiva valued the traditional approach to yoga teachings, she found herself "listening for a more integrative practice," and was drawn to studying with teachers who left a particular tradition or form and evolved their own way.

In her classes and teacher trainings, she sees an organic unfolding of the principles of the Krishnamacharya lineage, Tantric hatha yoga, and Ayurveda. "It's not so much about developing teachers that are all sharing the same style, but learning a set of tools for teaching that have very grounded principles for evolution." Her style emphasizes working from the simple to the complex, being able to see patterns in the body and then using the tools of yoga to unfurl those patterns. "Vinyasa means evolution, like a cycle. And flow is another way of describing Shakti, something that has this intelligent inherent rhythm and dance to it."

Shiva honors the feminine in her classes by choosing asanas that have more round, arced, and curvy shapes, which she explains is one of the ways in which Shakti moves. "It's like the water element associated with the moon in the feminine . . . there is a meandering shape to it, versus something like Virabhadrasana III (Warrior III pose) that is very linear and powerful in that linearity." When Shiva does teach the warrior series of poses, she invites her students to find the fluidity within the structure. In this way, Shiva feels we can move out of our habitual patterns and preserve the diversity of movement as an expression of Shakti by not getting stuck in the "frontal plane." Most of us live in the front of our bodies and need to move into our back bodies. Getting unstuck here helps us move out of our deeply etched patterns. Instead of rigidly sticking to a routine, she also encourages playing with the rhythm of your practice, slowing it down when the movement starts to get ahead of the breath—when it feels like an imposition rather than a dance between movement and breath.

"I think a lot of women need to feel a way to be in their strength that is nurturing. To be in their strength in a way that serves life and that doesn't masculinize their nervous system or their body." In her classes at Sacred Movement in Los Angeles, there is an equal ratio of men and women among the students. She emphasizes the "feminine" value of maintaining a relationship between the masculine and feminine principles, so that even though the practice may be particularly active and intense at times, students are "always bowing to the source of where that comes from."

Recognizing that other women struggle with issues of finding their own way in their yoga practice, in 2003 Shiva assembled a Yogini Conference at the Omega Institute to bring women together. "The reflection of the feminine way of practicing is not apparent. It's a naturally intuitive practice, but it shouldn't be such a lonely experience to come to that." The conference is now an annual event. Seeing women in her classes afraid to let their tears flow, or whose stomachs are so tight due to the cultural ideal of having a flat belly, has given Shiva some perspective on her own earlier experiences of branching out from the ashtanga system. "I look back and realize that I was attaching myself to the pole and I wasn't even chained. . . . I think that a lot of women feel this disapproving patriarchal authority that is ready to discount the intuitive way of knowing, because it hasn't been approved by 'His Holiness Shankaracharya' or something. Like we can't even name this thing that oppresses us." She describes going to temples in India and seeing hundreds of drummers and ecstatic devotees dancing as part of their spiritual practice. "No one can tell me what is part of yoga and what is not." Shiva sees this as a sacred time to heal the "spiritual snobbery" that demands outer credentials; a time to return to the essence of being.

While Shiva honors tradition, she pushes the envelope toward evolution and innovation. Because she conducted anthropological research while working on her master's degree at UCLA in the mid-'90s and has lived in Africa, the Caribbean, Nepal, and India, Shiva is familiar and comfortable with the creative tension between orthodoxy and synthesis. Like the mystical poets she so admires, Hafiz and Rumi, and bhakti (devotional) yogis like Andrew Harvey, Shiva sees an underlying commonality within diversity. "In the shuffle there are these people who look across the horizon and recognize something about us," she says, "who are always looking for that essence as it pervades across all of creation. Like looking for that same spark, that same sound, and hearing it sometimes in the most shocking places, the most rabid places, the most wild places, and reflecting that back so that our distinctions and separations don't get too hardened."

Shiva sees her roles as teacher, mother, CD and DVD producer, and creator of a yoga clothing line all as living yoga. Shiva feels that the imprint of the unconditional love of her late mother has influenced her perspective on yoga as an expression of the goddess. Shiva had a deep connection with her mother. As a "daughter of the goddess," Shiva sees every manifestation of life as an expression of this feminine energy; she sees her own life path as serving the goddess, and trusting in the undercurrent, not "pushing the river," but waiting for things to unfold on their own rather than impatiently forcing them. It is "this process of feeling a seed inside you but really waiting for the right season and then the right way for it to manifest. Looking for the signs and seeing when certain things start to sprout with the grace. And then the hard work comes in terms of nurturing. Expect some obstacles!" A large part of the creative process for Shiva has been accepting her messiness. She remembers looking at her vagina after birth, "Nobody ever talks about the way your yoni looks after birth. I mean it's beautiful, it's swollen, bloody, crusty—wow. If I am going to bring a creative energy into the world, I am going to have to get used to seeing that there are some natural places for chaos."

SHIVA REA, nationally renowned yoga leader and teacher trainer, is known for bringing the roots of yoga alive for modern practitioners through the integration of movement meditation, yogic philosophy and art, nature's vitality, spontaneous humor, and joy. She is a leading teacher of vinyasa flow yoga worldwide, writes for *Yoga Journal*, and lives with her family in Los Angeles, where she teaches at Exhale Center for Sacred Movement and UCLA's World Arts and Cultures Program. Shiva is the creator of several home-practice CDs, videos, and DVDs. www.shivarea.com.

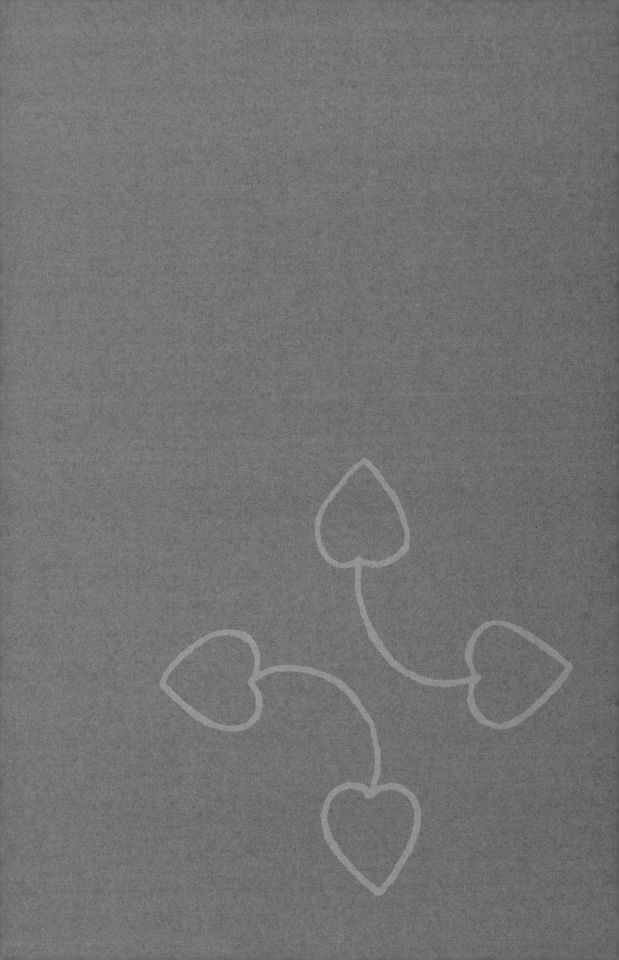

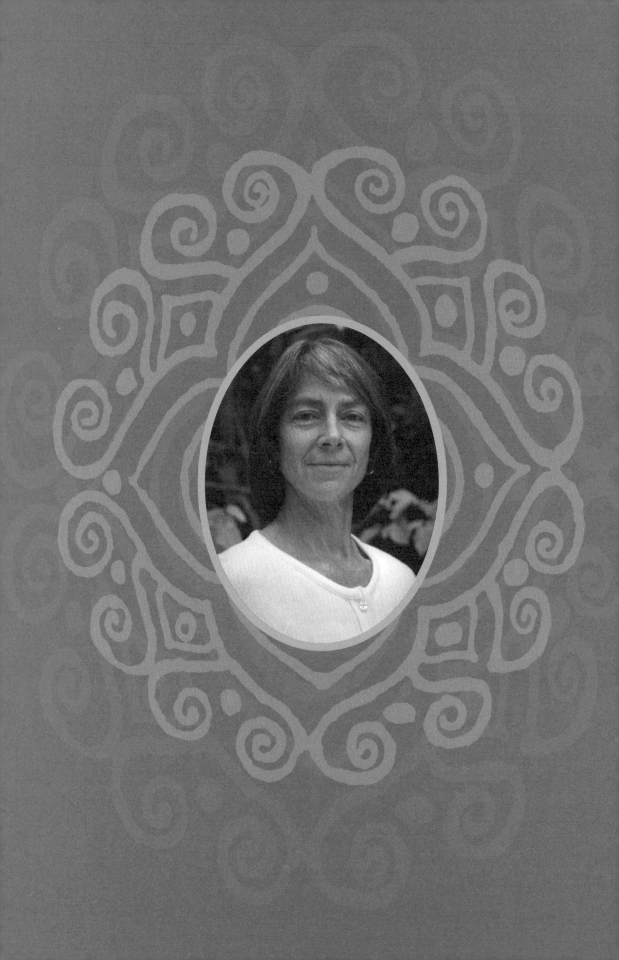

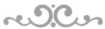

PATRICIA SULLIVAN

I'll study, I'll learn, I'll know.
It doesn't always quite go in that sequence.
Sometimes you have to fall down and
reexamine things and be willing not to know.

The Hindu goddess sensually poised on the altar in the studio where artist and yoga teacher Patricia Sullivan teaches commands a second look. The statue with multiple arms beckons the observer to come closer. On the left side, which is lean and muscular, a snake wraps around a thick ankle; on the right side, delicate jewelry adorns a round and voluptuous form. Is this figure male or female? A god or goddess? It is both. Shiva, the universal masculine principle, and Shakti, the universal feminine principle are united into one form, representing integration and balance. Together they symbolize the interplay of life and death, creation and destruction, form and emptiness. "She is incomplete without him and he is incomplete without her," Patricia says of this half-male, half-female deity that she herself sculpted. Drawing on her thirty-six years of yoga and meditation practice, she invites us to move beyond our conditioned ways of perception to unify what polarizes us and to recognize our innate wholeness. Through her teaching and her art, Patricia inspires us to look more deeply into our own nature.

Patricia's clay sculptures reflect the alchemical process of inner transformation through art, spiritual practice, and life. In 1984, the shapes of the yoga postures she had been practicing for fifteen years started to emerge when she was working with her potter's clay. These finely detailed figures of muscle, skin, and bone reflected her time studying Iyengar yoga and the anatomical body. In the early 1990s, when Patricia began studying Zen Buddhism and Tibetan yoga, she grew attracted to the female deities from the Hindu and Buddhist traditions, and they started taking form on her potter's wheel. "Everything is round when you throw it on a potter's wheel; that makes these pieces very feminine." The voluptuous goddesses she sculpts are physically the opposite of Patricia, who is angular and thin. "They're just round and I loved it. I thought, they can help me have this feeling of roundness and femininity and power.

They're not lacking in power for all their softness and roundness and femininity." It's clear that whatever Patricia makes, she ponders its deeper meaning; she feels her sculptures serve two purposes: they are an expression of some aspect of herself she needs to learn about or manifest in the world, and they are also for others to see what it calls forth in them.

While working on the Shiva-Shakti sculpture, also known as Ardhanarishvara, which means "half-woman," Patricia realized that the unification of male and female requires some destruction. "And who is Shiva? He is the lord of destruction and death, so here I am evoking the energy of destruction into my life." It took her over two years to create this piece. She dropped it several times and kept setting it aside because of this. At the time, she was going through the breakup of a twenty-year relationship, selling her share of the house, and giving up her yoga studio of nine years. Patricia felt like she had lost faith in something; she didn't know how to trust herself anymore, what direction to choose, where to live, where to teach.

Only one thing remained constant: "I hadn't lost faith in myself or any of my practices. I've stayed with my practices and my practices have stayed with me." But she realized that she had lost faith in the expectations instilled in her from childhood. Like many other women of her generation, she absorbed a host of messages as a young girl. The loudest one? That she needed to snag the "right" man. The expectation that she marry was built right into her name. While her brothers were given middle names at birth, she was not, as that would be provided by her maiden name after she married and took the name of her husband. Although she chose a less traditional path after finding yoga in 1970 at the age of twenty, part of her remained tethered to this unconscious plan. "And who is Shakti? There is nothing that can manifest without her. So, if something is going to happen, I am going to have to call on my feminine. And all my life I thought I was going to have to call on the masculine." Through her own search for wisdom and deeper understanding, Shiva-Shakti, this archetypal image of integration, came to life.

Patricia describes her first experience with consistent meditation practice as "exquisite relief" from doing yoga postures, "because I wasn't having to adjust or make it better . . . I just had to sit there and appreciate the silence." During the twenty years she lived, studied, and taught with Zen priest Edward Espe Brown, her understanding of the meditation process deepened. "To understand the sweetness and the peacefulness through mediation is very good. But, that, in my opinion, is preparation for what comes next, which is for all the difficulties to arise." But meditation is not invalid just because it calls up things that don't feel peaceful and joyful. "So you're there and you're breathing and you're with the essence of being; something arises and you put it down. But actually, there are many things that you need to pick up and deal with, so it's not all about putting it down. As Suzuki Roshi, a Zen teacher, used to say 'If you can't put it down, pick it up.'"

Patricia says she has never taken the easy path of letting someone else tell her what to do. "That path either hasn't worked for me, has harmed me, or hasn't stimulated me to go to the places I want to go." She spent twenty years studying and teaching yoga in the Iyengar tradition, following the lead of her teachers, who encouraged students to push through their limitations. At a certain point she realized that this wasn't what she wanted. She began questioning what it means to be a student and a teacher. She stopped studying with other teachers and began investigating through the laboratory of her own body. As a result, she started to hear her own voice emerging in her teaching. But there was another voice inside her, too, that told her that she didn't know enough, she wasn't good enough, and she needed to get the answers from someone else.

"If I always have to look to another teacher, look in a textbook to present something, how can I take enough authority to teach?" Patricia went through a period of time when she wasn't sure what voices to trust. "And that's a scary place to be, because what if my own voice doesn't have anything to say right now?" Coming up against the discomfort of walking into a classroom and feeling unsure of what and how to teach, even with decades of teaching experience, was both unsettling and transforming. "The assumption that 'I'll study, I'll learn, I'll know' . . . It doesn't quite go in that sequence. Actually, I think you have to fall down and reexamine things and be willing not to know." Patricia feels these old voices that get internalized can be replaced by new voices. "They're always going to be there, but if there are stronger voices with different things to say, they are going to be heard." She ultimately came to a place where the validity of her teaching was reflected in her own life and in her students' feedback.

Like the Divine Inspirator, a sculpture of the warrior goddess Durga she created, Patricia embodies a graceful strength that invites us to look into the nature of reality and into our true selves with compassion, honesty, and clarity. Just as she has done herself, Patricia reminds people to listen inwardly, to hone their attention, and tune in to not only the physical body but to the sensations, feelings, and emotions that are present. "We're raised in a society where we are taught that these levels of our being are not connected, and that we're not connected with each other." Rather than giving strong adjustments, she invites students to discover for themselves how much effort is truly needed to go into a pose. Patricia found that most people don't need a strong physical push, and that often when they are put into a pose by the teacher, it creates an expectation that they should be able to get there again on their own—setting up a cycle of expectation and disappointment. Now she educates teachers to increase their sensitivity to the energetic aspects of the practice. "If all your training is in asana, as most of mine had been, then you don't tend to open yourself to other kinds of perception."

Through challenges like a torn bicep, recent knee surgery, and relying on others for help through her separation, she has opened to an even deeper understanding of her own nature. "How can I be vulnerable without interpreting that, to myself, as weak? To be vulnerable is to be open. When I'm vulnerable, I'm not trying to prove anything, so I can just be more honest." Today, she feels that as her students see her as being vulnerable, it gives them permission to be vulnerable too. "And this whole world needs to lighten up with respect to being vulnerable. That's putting us in deep trouble. We all want to make our own little nest, our own little fortress, and then we're willing to let our leaders do what they're doing . . . I mean we're all in this together. Most of us would like to do something differently about it, and don't know where to start." For Patricia, the place to begin is right here with our relationship to our lives.

Patricia begins each day with prayer. "First, I speak my name, a powerful practice in itself. Then I describe my situation for this moment, for today, and I speak about all the factors that I can see or feel in this moment, often surprisingly self-revelatory. I don't know what will come up as I speak, so I learn something about my hopes and fears, about what I need and want." She then acknowledges the person she learned the ritual from, establishing a link to the ritual's tradition. Next, she speaks or sings her gratitude for the presence of spirit in her life and gives gratitude for the guidance, protection, and compassion she feels from this spirit. For this ritual, she uses floral water made in Peru. Water demonstrates a sensitivity to music, words, and intention. Words like *love* and *gratitude* have been found to transform water into beautiful snowflake-like crystals, while negative words, such as *hate* and *fear* make the water dark, amorphous, and without clear crystalline formations. Patricia smells the water and then anoints herself with it. "I feel quite empowered by this ritual, as I sing gratitude into the floral water every day and then put it on my body." She points out that if we don't have a way to reveal to ourselves what's important deep down within ourselves, we forget. "We get caught up in accomplishing and asserting our identity," she laughs out loud. "We forget that it changes every moment."

PATRICIA SULLIVAN began her yoga practice in 1970, and has been teaching since 1976. With roots in the Iyengar tradition, Patricia has carved out her own unique approach to yoga. In her teaching, she guides students towards greater sensitivity about the results of our actions on body, mind, and spirit, both in the context of the yogic practices and in daily life. Patricia's classes include chanting the yoga sutras of Patanjali, Vedic chants, asana, alignment work, pranayama, and meditation. Her work as an artist and sculptor also informs her teaching.

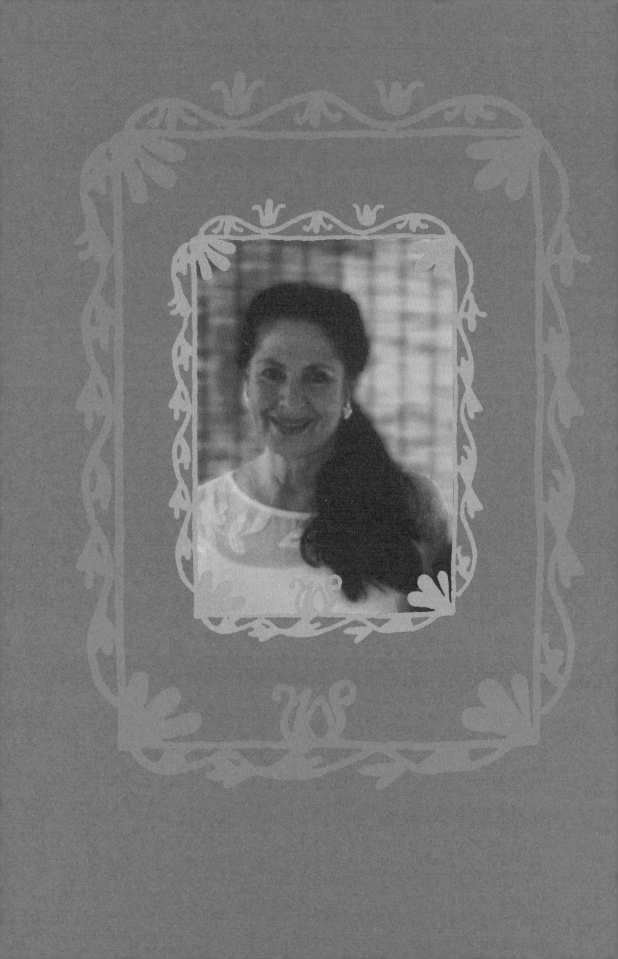

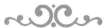

RAMA JYOTI VERNON

*Find the mountaintop in the
marketplace...stay in the world, transform
the world into the replica of the world
you're trying to get to. This is a very
different concept than
realizing the world is an illusion
and getting out of it.*

A t first glance, Rama Jyoti Vernon—with her mane of dark hair, ruby lips, and voluptuous curves—looks more like Sophia Loren than a diplomat for global peace, scholar, mother of five, and grandmother. A prolific creator, her first child was born when she was eighteen years old and her fifth at the age of forty-seven. Throughout her life, she's continued to give birth to many ideas and organizations; she seems to flow gracefully from one organization to the next, one side of the world to the other. She initiated the California Yoga Teachers Association and *Yoga Journal* magazine at her kitchen table. She organized the first yoga conference that brought together teachers from different traditions, Unity in Yoga. Her work in yoga and conflict resolution has taken her to Russia, the Middle East, Ethiopia, China, Central America, Ireland, Africa, Yugoslavia, and the inner cities of America. "The great thing about being a mother is that I really learned to let my children go," she says, "to follow their own path, without trying to superimpose my image on them, how they should live, what they should do." In the same way, she always knows when it's time to withdraw from an organization so it can continue to grow. "We have the Brahma,

Vishnu, and Shiva of the organizations: the creator, the sustainer, and the destroyer. I realized I am not a maintainer, I'm a creator. I really wanted that child to go on and to grow bigger and stronger."

Born into a pioneering family of natural healers, Rama was exposed to religion and spirituality since she was about four or five, through the Church of Religious Thought, where Ernest Holmes was her teacher. "We learned about how the mind has power over the body and that 'thoughts held in mind produce after their kind.' I studied that meditation when I was little, learning how to heal my own pains." Her parents ran a naturopathy school in their home. Her father, born in 1884, was one of the first chiropractors in the United States, and was instrumental in getting chiropractors recognized and granted licenses to practice as health professionals in California. Rama's mother, a physical therapist and surgical nurse, was one of the first reflexologists in the nation. "There were a lot of pearls that I gleaned from my mother and father. I feel so fortunate to have had the parents that I had. So I'm carrying on their work."

Rama's mother took her to her first yoga and breathing class when she was fifteen. "It was for people who were recovering from heart attacks and it was with an eighty-four-year-old Sikh master. He stood on his head and he did all the poses at eighty-four. I just sat there in disbelief." Rama studied pranayama as a teenager, but didn't study asana until she was twenty-two. Although she had parents who worked in the health field, she was a sickly child. She had arthritis, bronchitis, and a weak heart. "What yoga did was rearrange my whole cellular structure. I don't think I'd still be alive today if it weren't for yoga." With a deep calling to serve, she found that yoga was the missing link. "I loved religion. I was always searching for God. But I was so fatigued that I couldn't serve. I didn't have much to give to others. And then I discovered that combining asana, breathing, and meditation became a way to strengthen myself so that I could really serve others."

At twenty-seven, she began teaching yoga classes in her living room. Soon her classes were so big that she started training teachers, "so I could get a rest!" This growing body of teachers needed a way to communicate, so Rama started a newsletter, *The Word*, which eventually grew into *Yoga Journal*. To expand her teachers' knowledge and wisdom base, Rama began hosting workshops and bringing in teachers from different traditions, including Swami Vishnu-Devananda, Swami Satchidananda, and several Tibetan teachers.

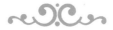

During this time, she was given BKS Iyengar's book, *Light on Yoga*. She could barely believe that the same person doing the poses had written the philosophy. "It was everything that I had discovered: that you cannot separate the poses from the other factors." She went to India to seek him out and brought him to California to teach for the first time in the early 1970s, when he was still unknown in this country. Only thirty people showed up; the next year, 125 came. As interest grew, Rama helped to start what eventually became the Iyengar Yoga Institute of San Francisco. When Iyengar wanted to implement a teacher certification program, he sent Rama to London to observe how it was being done there. "I went into the restroom and sobbed because I knew yoga before this. All of a sudden it was about the way they turned their kneecap, the way they turned their foot. Not about what was in the teacher's heart." She couldn't understand how things had gotten so far off track. "When I was in classes, Iyengar used to talk about philosophy a lot. And then he got away from it. Many people don't know what a deep mystic he was." After eight years, she left that community. "I'm a very strong, individual person. I just had to do my own thing. I think we all do, eventually. I didn't want to be bound by rules, because I had to let the spirit speak through me, move through me."

In 1983, while the Cold War still raged, Rama went to Russia, and it changed her life. "I went over there and I saw the enemy image that I had been conditioned to believe in. But I also saw the human being behind the façade, and they felt it. They opened their hearts to me." She decided to bring thousands of Americans over to meet their Soviet counterparts, to dissolve stereotypes and realize their similarities. "It was the greatest *sadhana* (spiritual practice) I've ever done." Subsequently, Rama was invited to develop dialogue forums and create peace exchanges between the two countries. Rama and her colleagues brought people together to build schools, birthing clinics, and hospitals through an organization called Social Inventions for the New Millennium, which developed over 1,000 joint projects between the two countries in healthcare, economics, the environment, education, spirituality, and the arts. They also arranged for American women to build the first peace wall in the middle of Moscow. "Just trying to find ways to keep the doors open," Rama comments.

This work expanded into the Center for Soviet-American Dialogue, a nonprofit group Rama created that brought her to Azerbaijan, which was at war with Armenia at the time. With a team of people from both countries, she helped facilitate peace talks. As the dialogues expanded, Rama realized that her work had evolved into conflict resolution.

When one of the ambassadors in Moscow asked her what she did that worked, she realized she was practicing the Yoga Sutras. No matter what country she visited or what leader she met with, it was all yoga. "Yoga has taught me that there is no separation."

Back in Washington, D.C., Rama met a Lebanese refugee named Marian, whose sole possessions were the clothes on her back. She had given up on the possibility of peace in the Middle East. When Rama talked to her about what she could do in the Middle East, Marian said there was nothing anyone could do. Rama held her hand as she cried. "She had such a hard life. I thought, how can I tell her that there's always something we can do? How can I tell her to think positively? How can I tell her you've got to hold a vision, when I haven't been through the experience that she's been through, where I lost everything?"

As a result of this meeting, Rama decided to bring together a group of women from Iraq, Lebanon, Israel, Palestine, and Iran so they could share their personal stories and their visions of peace. "The Israeli woman spoke about serving in the army, and then the Palestinian woman spoke of being on the opposite side of the army. And as each woman spoke, they broke down and cried, and I found that they were in each other's arms and they were holding each other. I sat there just astounded at the power of women sharing who they are." This idea grew and evolved, and Rama was asked to organize groups in Los Angeles, Chicago, New York, and Seattle. Before long, she began facilitating women across the country, in groups of fifteen to sixty. "They spent the whole day together and they went to such deep places . . . they shared their positive visions. Some of them said they felt they were floating on a cloud for two weeks after."

Inspired by the program's success and by the desire of these women to meet one another, Rama created a conference where they could gather. The first one, called Women of Vision: Leadership for a New World was held in 1994 in Washington, D.C., which eventually became Gather the Women. Rama worked with other pioneering women during this period, such as Barbara Marx Hubbard, Marian Williamson, Marilyn Ferguson, and Louise Hay. During these conferences, groups of women all over the world linked up in prayer and meditation on the same day at the same time, adjusting their time zones so that at the same moment everywhere women would "meet." "We held the vision of the world we wanted to see. Rather than focusing on what we didn't want, I thought, why don't we focus on what we want?" This concept was so powerful that in 2003, there were 405 simultaneous gatherings in twenty-three countries and

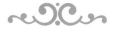

thirty-eight states dedicated to calling forth the feminine principle. Jean Shinoda Bolen, who was at one of these gatherings in Ireland, says the experience inspired her recent book, *Urgent Message from Mother: Gather the Women, Save the World*.

One day, while Rama was meditating, a voice told her that it was time to go back to teaching yoga teachers, which she did. "If you surrender and you offer yourself up as an instrument of service, then you have to go and do what you are being led to do." She created the American Yoga College in Tucson, Arizona, now known as the International Yoga College.

In 2004, Rama was called again to international work for the widows and orphans in Afghanistan. She has been exploring the possibility of creating a women's conference with representatives from Afghanistan, Iran, Iraq, Pakistan, Russia, and Turkey, and has met with female journalists, educators, and members of governmental ministries who are active in rebuilding their own countries. When teaching yoga to groups of Islamic women in Kabul, she explained that yoga meant "union." One woman asked, "Union with what?" Bridging their cultures with her words, Rama responded, "Union with God."

Over time, the divisions of her inner work and outer work in the world have blurred. "I found that I could no longer draw lines of demarcation, but found that one would support the other, and both were mutually interdependent." Today, Rama and her husband, Unity Minister Reverend Max Lasfer, teach an extensive curriculum in conflict resolution that reflects this understanding. The program, called From Individual to Global, is based on East-West psychology and explores the relationship between personal conflict and global conflict and how both can be transformed and used as a force toward positive change.

Ever the visionary, Rama's next endeavor is the International Peace College. "I've heard them talking about the war college for years, and I said that's enough, we've got to have a peace college." Currently, she is working with other educators on the development of a curriculum based on the Yoga Sutras. The program's three phases include the personal, the interpersonal, and application, where students travel into a country where they can apply the work. "When I say apply, it's not so much doing it with other people, it's applying it within themselves, from what they're observing. Can they hold two points or moral perspectives simultaneously without making one right and the other wrong? And that's from the yoga world."

Rama feels yoga now is coming forth as service. "At one time, that wasn't the original intent, which was withdrawing from the world. Now we're using it to be in the world and help change the world. It's like being the peace we want to see in the world. How can we want nonviolence around us when we don't have nonviolence within us? So, it doesn't do any good to get out of it, but like a *bodhisattva*, vow to be here and be the guide for others who have forgotten."

RAMA JYOTI VERNON has been at the forefront of the East-West yoga movement for over thirty-five years. She is a global peace diplomat, founder of six nonprofit organizations, including the Center for International Dialogue (CID, www.cfid.org), the International Yoga College (formerly American Yoga College), and *Yoga Journal* magazine. Her work with CID recently took her to Afghanistan to provide aid to women and children. Rama's Yoga Sutra–based work provides a unique approach to teaching national and international conflict resolution.

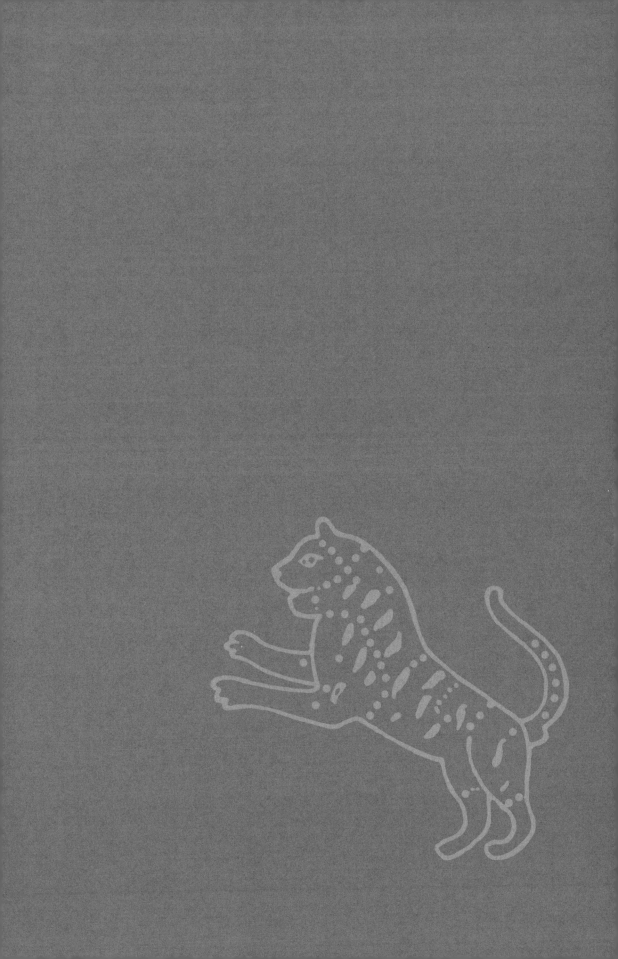

Luminaries

We all come from the Mother

and to Her we shall return

Like a drop of rain

flowing to the Ocean.

–Zsuzsanna E. Budapest

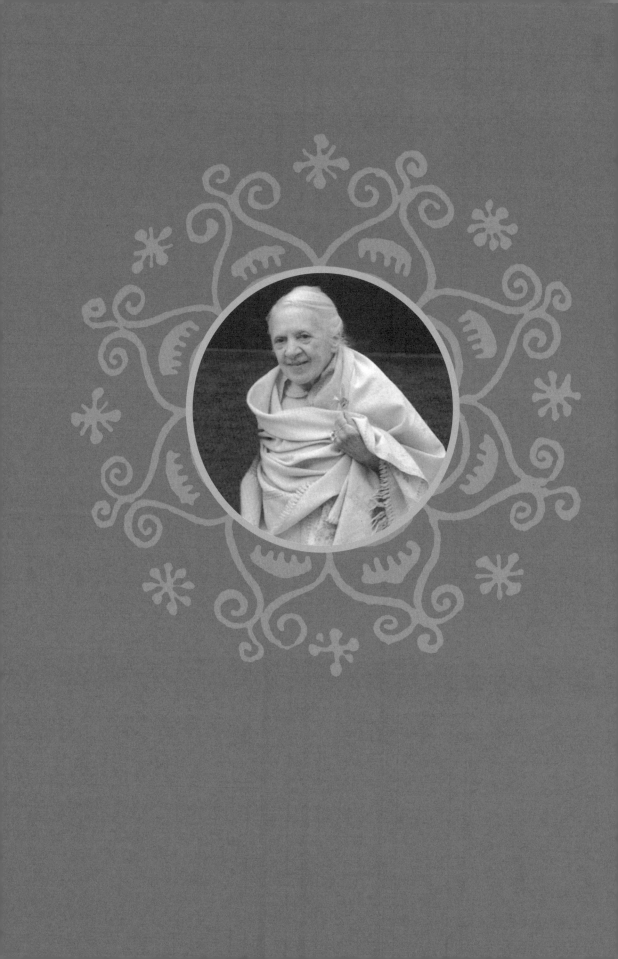

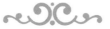

INDRA DEVI

1899–2002

We women must listen to our inner voice.
It is easier for women to do this,
as they are not afraid to say what they feel.
We must keep both our femininity
and our strength. Men have to descend from
their pedestal and learn how to be more
broad-minded and spiritual.

Born Zhenia Labunskaia in pre-Soviet Latvia in 1899, Indra Devi had a powerful influence on the spread of yoga throughout the Western world. Known fondly as Mataji (mother), her life and teaching spanned most of the twentieth century. After fleeing Latvia for Berlin with her mother in 1920, when the Communists invaded, Devi toured Europe with a theater group, as an actress and dancer. She was drawn to Indian culture and spirituality through the works of J. Krishnamurti and Madame Blavatsky, which eventually led her to India in 1927, where she continued acting (her name comes from a role in an Indian film). From that time on, she wore a traditional Indian sari and later became the first Western woman known to teach yoga in its country of origin.

In India, she married Jan Strakaty, a Czechoslovakian diplomat who was close friends with the Mysore royal family. As a guest at the Mysore palace for a wedding, Devi observed yoga classes taught under the direction of master teacher T. Krishnamacharya. This sparked her interest and she asked the king if she could attend the classes. The king insisted she could, although Krishnamacharya was unsure of her intentions. He tested her commitment by having her follow a strict diet and a schedule of twice-daily yoga practice. They quickly became close, and after a year, he encouraged her to teach.

When her husband was reassigned to Shanghai in 1939, Devi went with him and opened the first yoga school there. After World War II, she returned to India and wrote her first book, *Yoga: The Technique of Health and Happiness*. The book—and its sequel, *Forever Young, Forever Healthy*—became bestsellers, were translated into ten languages, and sold in twenty-nine countries. In 1947, her husband died and she moved to Hollywood, where she taught celebrities like Gloria Swanson, Greta Garbo, Marilyn Monroe, and the violinist Yehudi Menuhin. In 1953, she married Dr. Sigrid Knauer, a physician who bought her a beautiful eighty-acre ranch in Tecate, Baja California, Mexico, that served as a home, yoga retreat, and teacher-training center.

Fluent in five languages, Indra Devi continued to move easily throughout the world teaching yoga. Her conference for Kremlin functionaries led to the legal status of yoga in Russia; she is also credited with introducing yoga to China and Bulgaria, and has opened yoga centers in Mexico and Argentina. She fell in love with Argentina during a visit in 1982, so when her second husband died when she was eighty, she moved there, where she lived for the rest of her life.

Indra Devi taught up until a few years before her death in 2002, at the age of 102. Many loved her for her gentle, devotional approach to yoga, which she called Sai Yoga. Over 3,000 people attended her centennial birthday celebration in Buenos Aires. Her six yoga schools continue to offer daily yoga classes, and graduates from the four-year teacher-training program receive an internationally recognized college-level degree.

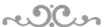

VANDA SCARAVELLI

1908–1999

It was only when I remained alone
that I discovered a new world in this field,
a world without aim and without competition,
where the body can start again and
again to function naturally and happily,
allowing expansion to take place.

Vanda Scaravelli was born in Florence, Italy, in 1908. The child of an artistic family, she was a classically trained pianist. As she grew up, she was exposed to a steady flow of intellectuals, artists, and scientists who visited her family, including Federico Fellini, Aldous Huxley, and the Indian philosopher J. Krishnamurti. As a girl, Vanda traveled with her family to Holland in search of spirituality and healing. When she grew up, she married a professor of philosophy and had two children. But it wasn't until midlife, in her late forties, that she discovered yoga.

When Vanda's husband died, shortly after World War II, she began spending summers with her children in Switzerland, where she rented a chalet and hosted Krishnamurti each year during his annual talks. BKS Iyengar came every morning to teach Krishnamurti yoga. Vanda had met Iyengar earlier, through her friend, the violinist Yehudi Menuhin, so when Iyengar was at the chalet, he gave Vanda private yoga lessons as well. She felt that yoga helped her survive this time of mourning. Several years later, at Krishnamurti's invitation, TKV Desikachar visited the chalet and introduced Vanda to the importance of the breath, which would become central to her teaching.

Soon Vanda felt the need for a less strenuous yoga practice, and began experimenting within the laboratory of her own body, finding ways to relax, unwind, and undo. Drawing on the anatomical precision she learned from Iyengar and Desikachar's emphasis on breath and ease, Vanda developed her own internal, intuitive approach to yoga. She focused on letting go of outer goals and worked with the natural movements of the body in relation to gravity—releasing and connecting to a deeper core energy that led to a spontaneous wave-like motion of the spine. Her willingness to surrender and trust in the wisdom of the body was reflected in her belief that yoga not be structured as a method, but discovered through each person's own experience. Her innovative approach influenced an entire generation of modern yoga teachers, including Angela Farmer, Dona Holleman, Erich Schiffmann, and Esther Meyers, who is most known for spreading Vanda's teachings.

The striking photographs of Vanda Scaravelli in her eighties—dropping her lean body into a backbend and wrapping herself into a ball with her feet crossed behind her head—are an inspiring complement to the text in her classic book, *Awakening the Spine*. Even more inspiring is the fact that she didn't start yoga until she was forty-five. Vanda died in 1999, at the age of ninety-one. Her fluid form can be seen in the video *Vanda Scaravelli on Yoga*, narrated and produced by Esther Meyers.

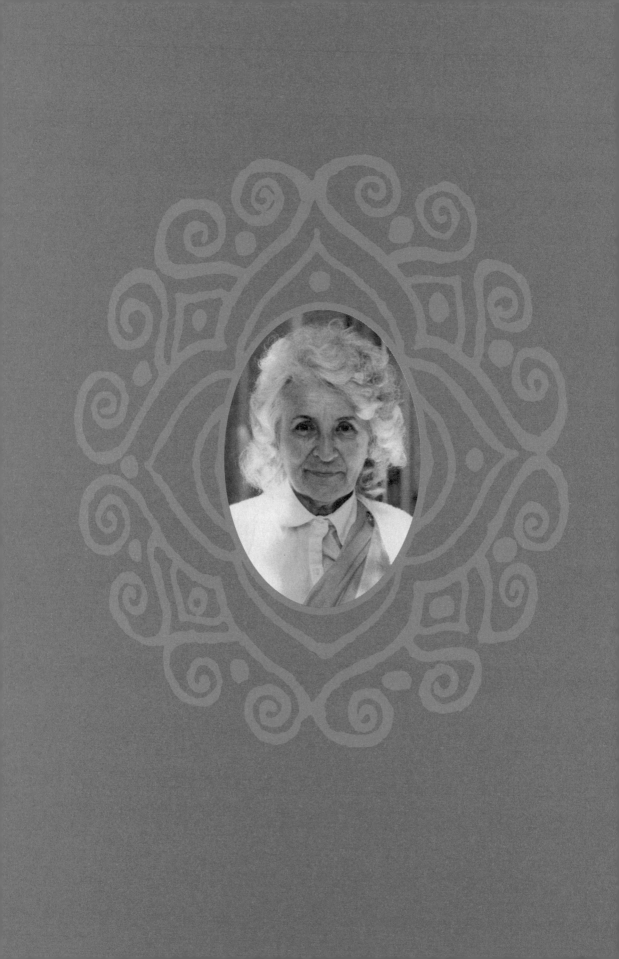

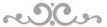

SWAMI SIVANANDA RADHA

1911–1995

In the Eastern tradition,
you are a discoverer,
an adventurer, and you become
your own laboratory, making your own
investigations. It is up to each person
to think intuitively,
to investigate, to inquire.

Born Sylvia Demitz in Berlin in 1911, Swami Sivananda Radha was a successful dancer before she and her husband, Wolfgang, turned their energy towards helping the persecuted escape from Berlin during World War II. As a result, the Gestapo executed Wolfgang in 1942 for crimes against the state. In 1947, she married a composer named Albert Hellman, but after only eighteen months, he died suddenly of a stroke. These experiences taught her a great deal about the realities of human existence.

She moved to England in 1949 and two years later emigrated to Canada, settling in Montreal. During meditation one day, the man who would become her spiritual guru, Swami Sivananda, appeared to her and told her to come to Rishikesh, India, to study with him. She went. In 1956, she became one of the first Western women to be initiated into the sacred order of sanyas. A year later, at her teacher's request, she returned to Canada as Swami Sivananda Radha (radha means "cosmic love"), and spent the rest of her life passionately committed to spreading the teachings of yoga. Through yoga, she was able to transform her early experiences into an understanding and compassion that lent great authority to her teaching.

One of the first female Westerners to bring yoga to the West, Swami Radha opened Sivananda Ashram Vancouver in Burnaby, British Columbia; in 1963 it was renamed Yasodhara Ashram and relocated to its present location on Kootenay Bay in the Canadian Rockies. Today it hosts a thriving spiritual community where people from all over the world come for workshops and retreats, and to learn about Swami Radha's teachings, which center around the practice of selfless service, or karma yoga. In 1969, Swami Radha created a journal for the ashram, *Ascent* magazine, which has blossomed into an international yoga magazine that connects yoga philosophy with the practical realities of daily living.

Known for her accessible teaching style, Swami Radha addressed issues of particular interest to women. In 1977, in a workshop entitled Women and Spiritual Life, she spoke about the purpose of life, how to live fully, and encouraged women to bring quality and light into their daily lives. She founded Timeless Books in 1978, through which she published twelve books based on teachings she received directly from Indian and Tibetan masters, her personal experience, and her own research on original texts. Her books include *Kundalini Yoga for the West*; *The Hidden Language of Yoga*; and *The Devi of Speech*, in which she writes about the connection between language and the creative forces of the divine feminine.

Inspired by her guru's request to spread the teachings, Swami Radha created a series of Radha Yoga Centers, opening the first one in Calgary in 1982. The Radha Yoga Centers now in the U.S., Canada, and Europe, offer classes in a supportive atmosphere for like-minded people seeking to deepen their self-knowledge. Swami Radha died in 1995, but the spirit of her work continues through her many centers, her books, *Ascent* magazine, and her successor, Swami Radhananda.

ACKNOWLEDGMENTS

i had no idea how much time and energy it would actually take when I declared that I was finally going to write this book. The gleeful madness that inspires and initiates all creative endeavors firmly took hold of me. Fortunately, as one of my teachers, Angeles Arrien, says, "Creativity is the fire that needs no wood." I bow to the source of that creativity for sustaining me throughout the journey of writing this book.

Many synchronistic events came together for this book to happen. I offer much gratitude to Jeff Klein, who has a knack for tuning in to what motivates people and developing their potential. At the end of a marketing consultation for my yoga studio, he asked just the right questions, inspiring me to resurrect this project. Within weeks, Jeff brought me to Mandala Publishing, where Acquisitions Editor Lisa Fitzpatrick "got it" right away: the time for this book was now. Thank you to Lisa for following your intuition and taking the leap of faith. My gratitude and appreciation to Nora Isaacs, my editor extraordinaire, who missed our first meeting because her baby, Lucian, decided to come into the world that day. Throughout the writing process, it seemed most appropriate to hear those sweet mothering sounds on the other end of the line during many of our phone conversations. Nora was the perfect fit for

this book and gave me essential guidance in writing. I also acknowledge Katherine Harper for her insight into the history of women in yoga and Linda Sparrowe for contributing the foreword.

It is due to the love and support of so many people that this book has actually come to fruition. I thank my soulful partner, Will Karnofsky, whose love and devotion is ever-present in my life, and without whose support and attentive care to our daughter I could never have done this. And to our daughter, Sacha Grace, who inspires me daily.

Writing a book takes to the extreme the phrase "it takes a village." My family has come through beyond the call of duty to engage my daughter while I spent more hours than I ever imagined I would sitting at the computer! A heartfelt acknowledgement to my mother, Patricia Duncan, for fortifying me with love and always trusting me to find my own way. And to my stepfather, Pete Duncan, for his love, support, and doting on little Sacha. And I am grateful to my father, Bob Gates, who always believes in me even when I don't, and was the first editor for many rough drafts. A thank you also to my stepmother, Deborah Welsh, for the extra support and insightful feedback.

Much gratitude to the rest of my family: my sister Laura Gates and her husband Laurence Polikoff—inexhaustible resources of support; my sister Nancy Gates for cheering me on from afar; Emily Kligerman—sister yogini; and Marv, Jeannine, and the rest of the Karnofsky clan.

A big thanks to my dear friends who continued to send their blessings when I vanished from sight: Rachel Adler, Anne Cushman, Liza Chapman, Nancy Evans, Robin Moody, and Lisa Nowell. And to my women's group for energetically holding me in the circle when I couldn't come in person. To Liisa O'Maley, my guardian angel, I am thankful for the books, the feedback, and her precious presence in my life.

Deep gratitude to my extended family at the Yoga Garden who make it such a special place: the teachers who kept things going while I was gone and enthusiastically covered my classes for me; Lisa Knowlton, who gave the studio extra attention and care in my absence; Catherine Henry, Elizabeth Weaver, and Lyman Spencer, who attend to numerous daily details. And I am grateful to the many students who continue to inspire me to do what I do, and who come to my classes and retreats year after year. I also want to acknowledge the wise teachers who have inspired my journey over the years: Amy Cooper, Angela Farmer, and many of the other women in this book. Thank you to the innovative yogi T. Krishnamacharya, through whose lineage of students I continue to learn so very much about yoga for healing. I offer my deepest appreciation to my sister-muse Nischala Devi and our teachers' circle for enriching this project in so many ways. I am eternally grateful to Deborah Chamberlin Taylor, Arina Isaacson, Athena Katsaros, and John Nicholas for their heartfelt guidance and mentoring. I offer a deep bow to the insightful dharma teachers at Spirit Rock and the Friday morning sangha.

Many thanks to Lisa Maria for her encouragement of my work; to Julie Rappaport and Kelly McGonigal for extremely valuable last-minute feedback; to Emilia Thiuri for overseeing the editing process, and to Jeanie Lerner for her thorough copyediting.

A special thanks to my first writing coach, Stephanie Moore, whose laser-like focus and high energy got me moving when I arrived with a pile of papers, completely overwhelmed. Her body didn't hold up to the ravages of cancer, but I could feel her fiery spirit guiding me daily.

I offer my deepest gratitude to the wise women in this book for taking the time to share their rich stories, experiences, and insights. And lastly, a heartfelt acknowledgement to the many women who don't appear in these pages—guiding lights in their own communities, everywhere.

— Janice

Bibliography

Note:
I drew great inspiration for the history from Katherine Harper, Professor of Art History at Loyola Marymount University, whose book, article, bibliography, and conversations were invaluable. I also relied heavily on the work of Vidya Dehejia as well as Georg Feuerstein's *The Yoga Tradition*.

Altekar, AS. *The Position of Women in Hindu Civilization*. Delhi: Motilal Banarsidas, 1962.

Dehejia, Vidya. *Devi the Great Goddess: Female Divinity in South Asian Art*. Washington DC: The Arthur M. Sackler Gallery, Smithsonian Institute, 1990.

———. *Yogini Cult and Temples*. Delhi: National Museum, 1986.

Dehejia, Vidya and Daryl Yauner Harnisch. *Representing the Body: Gender Issues in India's Art*. Delhi: Kali for Women, 1997.

Desikachar, Kausthub. *The Yoga of the Yogi*. Chennai, India: Krishnamacharya Yoga Mandiram, 2005.

Desikachar, TKV. *Health, Healing & Beyond: Yoga and the Living Tradition of Krishnamacharya*. New York: Aperture Foundation, 1998.

———. *Yogarahasya*. Chennai, India: Krishnamacharya Yoga Mandiram, Vignesha Printers, 1998.

———. *Yogayajnavalkya Samhita*. Chennai, India: Krishanamacharya Yoga Mandiram, Vignesha Printers, 2000.

Doniger, Wendy and Brian K. Smith. *The Laws of Manus*. New Delhi: Penguin Books, 1991.

Feuerstein, Georg. *The Shambhala Guide to Yoga*. Boston and London: Shambhala, 1996.

———. *The Yoga Tradition: Its History, Literature, Philosophy and Practice*. Prescott, Arizona: Hohm Press, 1998.

Findly, Ellison Banks. "Gargi at the King's Court: Women and Philosophical Innovation in Ancient India," in *Women, Religion, and Social Change*, edited by Yvonne Yazbeck Haddad and Ellison Banks Findly, 37-53. Albany: State University of New York Press, 1987.

Frawley, David. *Wisdom of the Ancient Seers, Mantras of the Rig Veda*. Salt Lake City, Utah: Passage Press, 1992.

Ghanananda, Swami. "Spiritual Tradition Among Hindu Women," in *Women Saints: East and West*, edited by Swami Ghanananda and Sir John Steward-Wallace, 1-8. Hollywood, California: Vedanta Press, 1979.

Gupta, Roxanne Kamayani. *A Yoga of Indian Classical Dance, The Yogini's Mirror*. Rochester, Vermont: Inner Traditions International, 2000.

Harper, Katherine Anne. "The Jina Mallia: Jainism and the Spirituality of Women." *Jinamanjuri: International Journal of Contemporary Jaina Reflections* 13 (1 April 1996): 42–63.

Harper, Katherine Anne and Robert L. Brown. *The Roots of Tantra*. Albany: State University of New York Press, 2002.

Johnsen, Linda. *Daughters of the Goddess: The Women Saints of India*. Saint Paul, Minnesota: Yes International Publishers, 1994.

———. *The Living Goddess: Reclaiming the Tradition of the Mother of the Universe*. Saint Paul, Minnesota: Yes International Publishers, 1999.

Kenoyer, Jonathan Mark. *Ancient Cities of the Indus Valley Civilization*. Oxford: Oxford University Press, 1998.

Leviton, Richard, "How the Swamis Came to the States." *Yoga Journal* (March-April 1990):41–55, 119–128.

Marshall, John. *Mohenjo-Daro and the Indus Civilization, Vol. I*. New Delhi: Asian Educational Services, 1996.

Mookerjee, Ajit. *Kali: The Feminine Force*. Rochester, Vermont: Destiny Books, 1988.

Olivelle, Patrick, trans. *The Upanisads*. New York: Oxford University Press, 1998.

Ramusack, Barbara N. and Sharon Sievers. *Women in Asia, Restoring Women to History*. Bloomington, Indiana: Indiana University Press, 1999.

Young, Katherine K. "Hinduism," in *Women in World Religions* edited by Arvind Shama, 59-103. Albany: State University of New York Press, 1987.

Shubhagana, Atre. *The Archetypal Mother*. Pune, India: Ravish Publishers, 1987.

Sjöö, Monica and Barbara Mor. *The Great Cosmic Mother: Rediscovering the Religion of the Earth*. San Francisco: Harper & Row, 1987.

Sparrowe, Linda with *Yoga Journal*. *Yoga*. Westport, Connecticut: Hugh Lauter Levin Associates, Inc., 2002.

Rieker, Hans-Ulrich. *The Yoga of Light: Hatha Yoga Pradipika*. New York: Seabury Press, 1971.

Yoga Journal. "'Yoga in America' Market Study," press release, February 7, 2005, available at: http://www.yogajournal.com/about_press020705.cfm.

Young, Katherine K. "Women and Hinduism," in *Women in Indian Religions*, edited by Arvind Sharma, 3–37. New Delhi: Oxford University Press, 2002

Young, Serenity. *An Anthology of Sacred Texts by and about Women*. New York: Crossroad Publishing Company, 1993.

Bibliography for Profiles:

Devi, Nischala Joy. *The Healing Path of Yoga*. New York: Three Rivers Press, 2000.

Durgananda, Swami. *The Heart of Meditation, Pathways to a Deeper Experience*. New York: SYDA Foundation, 2002.

Farhi, Donna. *Bringing Yoga to Life: The Everyday Practice of Enlightened Living*. New York: HarperCollins, 2003.

Folan, Lilias. *Lilias! Yoga Gets Better with Age*. New York: Rodale Books, 2005.

Gurmukh. *Bountiful, Beautiful, Blissful: Experience the Natural Power of Pregnancy and Birth with Kundalini Yoga and Meditation*. New York: St. Martin's Press, 2003.

Lasater, Judith, PhD, PT. *Living Your Yoga: Finding the Spiritual in Everyday Life*. Berkeley, California: Rodmell Press, 2000.

Ruiz, Fernando Pages. "The Feminine Critique." *Yoga Journal*, (July-August 2002): 141–143.

Scaravelli, Vanda. *Awakening the Spine; the Stress-Free New Yoga That Works with the Body to Restore Health, Vitality and Energy*. New York: HarperCollins, 1991.

NOTES

[1] Barks, Coleman, translator, *Naked Song: Lalla* (Athens, Georgia: Maybop Books, 1992), 64.

[2] Williams, Joanna, "The Construction of Gender in the Paintings and Graffiti of Sigiriya," in *Representing the Body: Gender Issues in India's Art*, by Dehejia, Vidya, and Daryl Yauner Harnisch (Delhi: Kali For Women, 1997), 65.

[3] Noble, Vicki, *Uncoiling the Snake: Ancient Patterns in Contemporary Women's Lives* (New York: HarperCollins, 1993), 132.

[4] Ghanananda, Swami and Sir John Steward-Wallace, *Women Saints East and West* (Hollywood, California: Vedanta Press, 1955), 3.

[5] Doniger, Wendy and Brian K. Smith. *The Laws of Manu* (New Delhi, India: Penguin Books, 1991), 124.

[6] Ibid., 5: 154, p. 115.

[7] Ibid., 9: 65, p. 205.

[8] Johnsen, Linda, *The Living Goddess* (Saint Paul, Minnesota: Yes International Publishers, 1999), 5.

[9] Mookerjee, Ajit, *Kali: The Feminine Force* (Rochester, Vermont: Destiny Books, 1988), 27.

[10] Barks, *Naked Song: Lalla*, 21.

[11] Ibid., 49.

[12] Hirshfield, Jane, ed., *Women in Praise of the Sacred: 43 Centuries of Spiritual Poetry by Women* (New York: HarperCollins Publishers, 1994), 138.

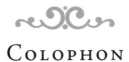

Colophon

Main body text was typeset in Adobe Jenson Pro, which was designed by Robert Slimbach of the Adobe type design team. Slimbach based it on Nicolas Jenson's roman and Ludovico degli Arrighi's italic typeface designs. The part openers and drop capital letters were typeset in Julia Book, designed by Jim Marcus.

Mandala Publishing

Publisher and Creative Director: Raoul Goff

Executive Directors: Michael Madden and Peter Beren

Acquisitions Editor: Lisa Fitzpatrick

Art Director: Iain Morris

Designer: Michele Wetherbee

Project Editor: Emilia Thiuri

Coordinating Editor: Nora Isaacs

Production Manager: Lisa Bartlett

Studio Production: Noah Potkin

Mandala would like to thank Jeff Klein, Carina Cha, Monika Lasiewski, and Nam Nguyen.

Photo & Illustration Credits

vi: Courtesy of Mahaveer Swami

vii: Courtesy of the Victoria & Albert Museum, London

4: Courtesy of B.G. Sharma

10: Borromeo/Art Resource, NY

13: Scala/Art Resource, NY

17: Courtesy of the Victoria & Albert Museum, London

18: Courtesy of Mahaveer Swami

21: Courtesy of Mahaveer Swami

23: Courtesy of Mahaveer Swami

26: Photograph courtesy of Kim Frances, sculpture by Patricia Sullivan

29: Courtesy of the American Institute of Indian Studies

31: Photograph of Sharon Gannon courtesy of Connie Hansen

36: Photograph of Nischala Joy Devi courtesy of Barbara Bingham

44: Photograph of Donna Farhi courtesy of Fred Stimson

52: Photograph of Angela Farmer courtesy of Victor Van Kooten

60: Photograph of Lilias Folan courtesy of Circe Hamilton

66: Photograph of Sharon Gannon courtesy of Connie Hansen

74: Photograph of Sally Kempton courtesy of Jim Needham

82: Photograph of Gurmukh Kaur Khalsa courtesy of Fran Gealer

88: Photograph of Judith Hanson Lasater courtesy of Judith Hanson Lasater

104: Photograph of Sonia Nelson courtesy of Cathy Maier Callanan

112: Photograph of Sarah Powers courtesy of Matthew Carden

120: Photograph of Shiva Rea courtesy of James Bailey

128: Photograph of Patricia Sullivan courtesy of Patricia Sullivan

144: Photograph of Indra Devi courtesy of Fondacion Indra Devi

148: Photograph of Vanda Scaravelli © Rob Howard

152: Photograph of Swami Sivananda Radha courtesy of Derek French